Hazardous To Your Health

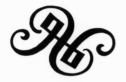

HAZARDOUS
TO YOUR HEALTH

A New Look at
the "Health Care Crisis" in America

MARVIN HENRY EDWARDS

ARLINGTON HOUSE   NEW ROCHELLE, N.Y.

RA
445
.E33

SECOND PRINTING, NOVEMBER 1972

Library of Congress Catalog Card Number 73-183679

ISBN 0-87000-138-8

MANUFACTURED IN THE UNITED STATES OF AMERICA

For Julie
Friend and colleague, as well as wife

Contents

Acknowledgments

In the usual manner of making such computations, this book has been some three years in preparation, and five months in the writing. But that is an inadequate measurement, for it is a count only of my own time, and there is far more than my own work in the pages that follow.

Wherever possible, I have indicated the source of the material I have used, and I have attempted to give full credit to the authors whose ideas and writings have contributed to my work. I gratefully acknowledge them here for the insight and understanding they have given me, and for their assistance, knowing or otherwise, in helping me prepare the evidence for the case I present.

In addition, there are many other persons who have contributed to this book in a variety of ways. If I were to thank each of them, this acknowledgment, traditionally brief, would constitute a chapter in itself. There are some, however, who must be mentioned.

I owe thanks to my good friend M. Stanton Evans, editor of the *Indianapolis News*, for leading me, first, to the editorship of *Private Practice* magazine, from which vantage point I have been able to observe the growing dangers of which I write in this book, and, secondly, for leading me to his friend David Franke.

And to David Franke himself, my ever-patient editor at Arlington House, for his good nature in dealing with a beginning author, and for his help in making the work presentable.

I owe thanks, also, to Barbara Landon, Nancy Jones and Mike Redwine of my staff at *Private Practice* for their constant help and encouragement, and to Myron Zimmerman of New York for his assistance in obtaining information that was invaluable in the preparation of this book.

I am deeply indebted to Professor Robert J. Myers of Temple University for his assistance in compiling the information presented in Chapter 10, and to Allan Brownfeld for the information he provided for Chapter 13.

I owe special thanks to Dr. George C. Roche III, President of Hillsdale College, and to Joan Hobson, of London, England, who has to live with the system we hope so desperately to avoid.

I could not let this opportunity pass without long overdue thanks to my colleagues on the board of directors of *Private Practice* magazine for the education they have given me and the patience they have shown with a new editor. They are: Joseph F. Boyle and Charles Johnson of Los Angeles; John Hawk of Charleston, South Carolina; Bob Knapp of Wichita, Kansas; Neal Flowers of Mobile, Alabama; Bill Haeck of Grand Rapids, Michigan; Frank Coulter of Kansas City; Lester Karotkin of Houston; Marshall Driggs of Englewood, New Jersey; Dick Frey and Tom Cook of Minneapolis; and Larry Tilis of Rochester, New York.

* * *

For more things than I can relate, I am especially indebted and grateful to my friend and, in many ways, my inspiration for this book, Dr. Francis A. Davis of Shawnee, Oklahoma.

Preface

This book is the result of a long series of assaults on reason that, over the past decade, has increasingly awakened in me a sense both of remorse and of crusading passion.

This is a book about medicine. Yet I am not a medical doctor. Nor am I, any more often than the ordinary citizen, in the position of being a patient. Why then does my alarm center now on the proposition that the United States shall adopt a system of national health insurance? Obviously, a socialized medical system is not the only precipice toward which our nation is headed.

The answer lies in the nature of medicine itself—or, at least, medicine as it has recently been practiced in the United States.

The practice of medicine is a personal thing, imbued with an intimacy found in few other areas of human life. Though supermarket chains and giant department stores are a large part of the free market system, it is the individual entrepreneur—the doctor, the small shopkeeper, the independent television repairman—who, in my opinion, lies at the base of that system of private initiative that has provided so well for the American people. Of all occupations, and especially of the professions, medicine, like the law, stands apart in its requirement of two essential characteristics of a free society—the right to privacy and the right of individuals to choose freely those persons with whom they will establish relationships of trust and confidence.

I have long been convinced, as I participated in discussions, attended (and gave) speeches, and generally participated in the political process, that if the American public could ever be persuaded to surrender to government any of those areas of concern that have for so long constituted the ultimate in *private* relationships, the drift of the nation into some form of impersonal and inefficient state socialism, with its strangling web of restrictions and regulations, would be immeasurably speeded.

As a newspaperman in the late 1950s and early 1960s, I had managed, for a time, to remain fairly well informed of the major issues of the day, but crises of government, encroachments upon personal liberties, and political assaults upon the free market system soon began to occur with such exhausting rapidity that all of them eventually became entangled in a hodge-podge of sameness. It was impossible to keep on top of all of them and adequately to distinguish the urgent from the less urgent to establish priorities (even if only priorities of personal concern).

Then, in the summer of 1968, M. Stanton Evans suggested that a group of doctors who were then forming a new medical journal ask me to be its editor. In September of that year I joined *Private Practice*, and thus began an intimate contact not only with the private medical system, but also with its critics, its reformers, detractors, and (in smaller numbers, at least in the press) its advocates.

I became attuned to the things that were happening, politically, to medical doctors and to their profession, and to the implications in those happenings for me, as a potential patient, and for the entire system of free enterprise in this country.

Because I am not a medical doctor, my concerns were not with the increased or decreased personal income that might result from government medical programs—concerns that may distract some MDs from the more significant aspects of their own problems. I was free, therefore, to view the problem from a somewhat different perspective.

This is *not* a pro-doctor book. There are doctors, as there are persons in every profession and occupation, who, for various reasons, endorse programs of government financing and government control, and who are unaware of the dangers in that course. Some doctors, in fact, might call this an *anti*-doctor book. Since 1965,

Federal health care programs such as Medicaid and Medicare have paid for patient services that were previously rendered free; doctors who have chosen to participate in these programs have sometimes been rewarded with increased incomes. Now they assume that if some government medicine is good (that is, financially good, for them), then more is better.

This is, instead, a pro-patient book. For if national health insurance or any of the broad-scale government health programs that have been proposed become law, it is the patient who will pay, in terms of higher medical costs (through increased taxation) and lower quality medical care.

And it is a pro-private enterprise book. For I am convinced now, more than ever before, that if government takes over the free-market medical system, it will soon take over far more.

Though I had accumulated a large amount of material about national health systems in the United States and other nations, and much material, also, about the true nature of the so-called "health care crisis" in this country, most of the material had been used solely for background information for my editorials in *Private Practice*, and as leads for feature articles that have appeared from time to time in that magazine. This book began, in my mind at least, in late 1970. A series of trips to Washington, D.C., resulted in my becoming aware that even those relatively few persons in the capital who devote themselves to a defense of the free-market system were largely unaware of the false nature of the "health crisis" propaganda to which they had been so frequently subjected, and of adverse ways in which a government-run health system would affect the quality, availability and cost of medical care in this country.

When Dan Joy, the editor of *The New Guard* magazine, asked me to prepare two articles on the subject, I found that the information I had compiled constituted a devastating indictment of government health systems, and a strong defense of private medicine in the United States. It was the preparation of those articles that led to the writing of this book.

The attempt to replace private medicine with a government health system grows in intensity each day. The *Washington Evening Star* has described the battle over national health insurance as the "political sizzler of the 70s." Yet there is no debate over the basic issue. It is assumed that *some* form of government health program is inevitable, and the question is simply: *Which* plan?

Every American, of whatever age, has a valuable stake in the preservation of the medical system that, for many years, has provided the great majority of citizens with high quality care at a relatively low cost. I am not so naïve as to believe that this book —alone against a tide of books that damn and condemn private medicine—will accomplish that task. It will serve my purpose if it merely helps to create the debate that is lacking, for I am confident that if the American people are given an opportunity to consider not the inevitability of some form of government medicine, but the question of whether they want government medicine at all, they will opt to keep instead the system that has served them so well.

Marvin Henry Edwards
Oklahoma City
June, 1971

PART ONE

THE CAMPAIGN

1. Goodbye, Marcus Welby

The latter half of the twentieth century may someday be remembered as the age of depersonalization—the era in which man was computerized, numbered, herded into mass-transit systems and stacked into one- and two-bedroom cubicles.

There has remained, however, one significant and cherished reminder of man's individuality—the face-to-face confrontation with his own private physician. Medical care, the most personal and intimate non-family relationship in present-day life, has remained essentially a private affair.

At least it has remained so in the United States. In nation after nation, private medicine has been replaced by the medicine of politics. America may be next.

This book is not about Marcus Welby, the fictional physician of national television, but it *is* about the grim possibility that, within the very near future, the style of medicine that Dr. Welby represents—personal, concerned, compassionate—will be replaced by a new and unfamiliar medical system—cold, impersonal, detached. The new system will render assembly-line care, with the patient having no choice in the selection of the doctor who will treat him, and the doctor having limited choice in the treatments he can render. And this mass medicine—imposed in the name of economy—will cost the American patient far more than he now pays to stay well.

This is the ominous prospect if the United States ignores the hard lessons to be learned from those countries that have adopted national health programs—countries that now have hundreds of thousands of patients waiting to get into hospitals; countries in which doctors lie and connive to find beds for their patients; countries in which doctors mass-treat thousands of patients, with only minutes available for each one; countries in which politicians debate mercy killings of the aged in an effort to reduce the massive cost of government medicine.

This is the grim prospect, in short, if the United States is led by the false propaganda of a "medical crisis" into a system of national health insurance. m

Is socialized medicine coming at last to America? It seems increasingly likely that it is. Although none of the proposals now before Congress specifically advocate socialized medicine—technically a system in which the state owns as well as controls the means of production—the differences are minute, and experience in other nations has clearly revealed the simplicity with which national health insurance systems can be converted into completely socialized medicine.

Whether socialized medicine or a major step toward it, national health insurance programs now before Congress will send the costs of health care soaring and seriously reduce the quality of the medical care patients receive in return.

Some idea of the sort of care that might follow creation of a national health system was revealed in early 1971 by Frank Furstenberg, a principal figure in the late Walter Reuther's Committee for National Health Insurance. Appearing in a televised debate sponsored by the American Enterprise Institute, Dr. Furstenberg envisioned a system in which government planners would provide a more ideal distribution of medical manpower, using midwives to deliver babies and thus free medical doctors for other duties.

Dr. Furstenberg speaks with some authority when he describes medical care under a system of national health insurance. The Committee for National Health Insurance, which he represents, drafted and sponsors the medical bill introduced in the Senate by Edward Kennedy.

It should come as no surprise that national health insurance might well herald the return of the midwife. Senator Kennedy, in his introduction to Daniel Schorr's polemic *Don't Get Sick in America,* publicly bemoaned the fact that the United States is the only major industrial nation in the Western world that has not adopted a compulsory nationwide government health system. In many of the nations he eyes with envy, most births are performed by midwives rather than physicians.

And, Senator Kennedy hints, national health insurance is to provide the "lever" for more drastic changes to come.

Increased cost and lower quality care are not the only dangers that flow from national health insurance. In an era of ever-shrinking areas of privacy, government health programs threaten to intrude into the most intimate aspects of a patient's life. The pattern, in fact, has already been set. A large number of Americans—military veterans, the aged and the indigent—are already treated in government health-care programs, and the bureaucracy has made its intentions clear.

In March, 1971, Louisiana Blue Cross, acting as an intermediary agent for the Department of Health, Education and Welfare, demanded that St. Joseph Hospital, in Thibodaux, release confidential medical records of patients who had applied for Medicare benefits. The hospital, clinging to codes of ethics prescribed by the American Hospital Association, American College of Hospital Administrators, Joint Commission on Accreditation of Hospitals, and the medical profession itself, refused. Although St. Joseph admitted the right of government agencies to inspect records that would prove whether or not the patient had actually received the treatments for which funds were claimed, it was *not* willing to release, as the government had demanded, confidential patient-interview files.

In an article entitled "The Fight for the Patient's Privacy," in the June, 1971, issue of *Private Practice* magazine, Allan Brownfeld described the sort of information contained in the files the government was seeking—information taken from an actual case history:

"Crying, pessimism, bleak future, tension, headaches, nervousness—indefinite period actually, but inclined to date everything from accident—lied to me at first, saying she hadn't been told a psychiatrist was called in, then inadvertently admitting it. Psychomotor retardation apparent. Unable to discuss more personal and intimate problems at this interview. I suggested she see me after discharge, but she said she'd snap out of it, which I doubt since the syndrome seems to be growing *worse* rather than better with the passage of time. She has taken an overdose of pills on one occasion and I think she needs psychiatric assistance, but she is not psychotic at this time and I know of no way to force her into treatment. . . ."

This patient was hospitalized for fainting at work. She claims Medicare reimbursement only for treatment she actually received —treatment verified by other, available, records. Because she accepts government money, the government declares it has the right to know the most intimate details of her life—details known only to her family and to her doctor.

The government is adamant. In separate letters, Thomas E. Jeffcoat, vice president of professional and governmental affairs for Louisiana Blue Cross; Irwin Wolkstein, assistant director of HEW's Bureau of Health Insurance in Baltimore; and Mrs. Martha A. McSteen, HEW's regional representative in Dallas, all declared that the government has a right to inspect the private records that doctors keep to help them treat their patients—records that doctors are ethically forbidden to reveal even to a patient's husband, wife, children, or parents.

Today, this intrusion by government investigators extends only to military veterans receiving government-financed treatment and to those unfortunate elderly or poor who, since 1965, have accepted government funds to meet their health care needs. Under a system of national health insurance, which extends Federal money to all Americans, all will become similarly subjected to bureaucratic invasions of medical privacy.

And, once national health insurance becomes law, if it does, there may be no way out for the helpless patient entrapped in the web of government waste, inefficiency and regulation. Or, at least, no feasible way out. Just as the advent of Medicare practically eliminated the availability of private medical insurance for persons over 65, national health insurance will effectively abolish all of the nation's private health insurance programs—programs which now cover nearly 90 percent of the population. In Britain, the deterioration of medical care under the nation's government health system has driven some two million persons back to the shelter of private insurance plans, but that is only four percent of the population—

not enough to support a highly competitive private insurance industry—and each must pay double for the privilege, once in private insurance premiums and again in the high taxes levied to keep the government program going.

(National health insurance will thus permanently close most private insurance companies and displace thousands of workers, but that is not the subject of this book.)

The planners' plans are not secret. Late in 1970, Robert J. Myers, chief actuary of the Social Security Administration since the Truman administration, resigned. Top Social Security officials, he said, believe the government should take over the provision of virtually all economic security for the entire population, thus eliminating private enterprise.

Why the vast nationwide campaign for national health insurance? And why the support for it? The answer is twofold.

First, national health insurance, like other broad-scale government social programs, has long been a cherished goal of those who carry the torch for that particular ideology that holds that it is the responsibility of government to care for, provide for, and, as a necessary consequence, control its nation's people.

It is an ideology both of paternalism and of arrogance, based on the sincere desire of some to provide for others, and the belief that the people are incapable of caring for themselves, and on an assumption of superiority that has consistently marked the claim by some of the right to regulate and direct others.

The second part of the answer is less complex: in an age when more and more people have become accustomed to the government handout—to receiving more from society than they have contributed to it—the promotion of social programs has become politically the thing to do.

Although early leaders of the labor movement opposed national health insurance, it has since become a favorite labor cause, primarily under the motivation of the late Walter Reuther. It has also surfaced, from time to time, as a major political vehicle—most recently for Senator Edward Kennedy, who in mid-1971 barnstormed the nation in a series of "health crisis hearings" that received widespread criticism, even from such liberal publications as the *Los Angeles Times* and from black politicians, as a purely political jaunt. (The hearings were "established to promote Senator

Kennedy, not to adequately research health care," complained an aide to Harlem's State Senator, Sidney Von Luther.)

Nonetheless, the campaign is underway and, fueled by a sudden rash of "health crisis" books, television "documentaries" and magazine articles, is escalating into the major domestic issue of the decade. But is it based on fact or on the myth of political propaganda? Is there a health "crisis" in the United States? What's behind the "spontaneous" campaign for a national health system? Will national health insurance cost less and improve medical care, as its advocates contend, or will it cost more—from both the government and the individual taxpayer—and reduce the quality of medical care? Will it fulfill its advocates' expressed desire for "high quality medical care for all," or will it prove hazardous to your health?

These are the things this book is about.

2. Medicine's Labor Pains

Andrew Biemiller is a former Wisconsin Congressman who was rejected by the voters in 1950, along with other liberal advocates of national health insurance. Today he is a lobbyist for the AFL-CIO. Biemiller has made it clear that organized labor, leader of the campaign for national health insurance since the death of Samuel Gompers, intends to have such a law soon.

Labor's drive has been relentless and has culminated in a recent rash of Congressional testimony, public statements and legislative string-pulling designed to force Senator Edward Kennedy's national health insurance proposal into law. Kennedy's bill is labor's grandchild. The bill itself is a creation of the late Walter Reuther's Committee for National Health Insurance. It won AFL-CIO support in 1971 after George Meany's amalgam of labor unions had entered its own bill—introduced by Representative Martha Griffiths—in the 1970 Congressional session.

Today the labor movement, headed by Reuther's United Auto Workers and the AFL-CIO, is the nation's leading campaigner for a change in the American medical-care system. Leonard Woodcock, who succeeded to the UAW presidency—and chairmanship of the Committee for National Health Insurance—on Reuther's death, is the campaign's leading spokesman.

Now, labor senses victory, and has gone in for the kill. "The need for action is urgent," Woodcock said in June, 1970, in a statement following his appointment to succeed Reuther. National health insurance, he said, is "inevitable."

Indeed, there are increasing indications that some form of national health insurance may be imminent, unless something is done soon to slow its advance. After more than half a century, the strident voices of labor leaders and professional left-wingers have been joined by those of more moderate supporters.

No matter what the cost of private medical care, advocates of national health insurance had contended that it was too high. No matter what the supply of physicians or the state of medical science, advocates of national health insurance had charged that physicians were too few and medical care inadequate. In recent years, however, they have found unforeseen help. Though medical-care costs continue to rise at a slower pace than many other living costs (see Chapter 5), government economic policies of the past decade have created a highly visible inflation, pushing all prices skyward. Along with the costs of food, housing, and transportation, medical costs have risen. With hospitals stricken by the same inflation—and by union demands that have forced construction costs upward and brought liberal pay increases to hospital employees—the costs of hospitalization have climbed rapidly.

An embittered public, finding it harder and harder to make ends meet, has become increasingly receptive to labor's criticisms of the medical system. Frustrated by the treadmill they find themselves on —and unable to do much about it—some people have begun to take up the liberals' line that "something must be done." So far the number who have fallen into the trap is comparatively small. Public and private opinion surveys have reported that the average American is still fairly well satisfied with his physician and the medical care he receives. Yet the frustration exists and the campaign—pursued daily through the media—is making some headway.

The first to fall in line have been members of the media themselves. Newspapers, television networks, and mass circulation magazines have begun to repeat the intonations and slogans, and have either called for national health insurance or simply contented themselves with the traditional cry: "Something must be done."

One of the first to join the attack was *Time* magazine. In a lengthy special report, in February, 1969, *Time* unleashed a bitter attack on health-care costs and "wretched" medical care. At times the criticism reached emotional depths of absurdity: "Theoretically," the magazine cried, "it would be possible for a man to have graduated from medical school at 25 in 1934, to have been licensed after a year's internship, and to have practiced as a GP ever since without having heard a professional word about most of modern medicine."

As stated, of course, the criticism was true. "Theoretically," a physician could practice in total isolation from the advances of medical science. But a 1969 survey of 3,200 Brooklyn physicians revealed that each doctor, on the average, spent 345 hours a year continuing his medical education by attending lectures and meetings, taking courses, and reading medical journals. That amounts to nearly one and a half months in eight-hour days—all after regular working hours.

Time's article charged, with no attempt at documentation, that three-fourths of all Americans get only "passable," poor, or bad medical care—a charge leveled at a time when life spans were increasing and infant illness and mortality rates were decreasing.

For page after page, *Time* continued its shrill rhetoric.

The people, *Time* said, were demanding to know the answers to a number of questions. For example, "Why did the doctor refuse to make a house call?" and "Did the doctor take too long in making the right diagnosis?"

Time did not, however, bother to present some of the obvious answers to those questions. Most doctors, for example, make house calls infrequently primarily because (a) if the description of symptoms indicates that immediate treatment is unnecessary, a house call will merely eat into the doctor's limited time—and add to the patient's medical bill—with no benefit in return, or (b) if the symptoms indicate that immediate treatment *is* necessary, proper care will usually require getting the patient to the doctor's office, or to a hospital, where the doctor will have available more modern equipment and medication than he can generally fit into his small black calling bag.

As for concern about the length of time spent by physicians in diagnosing their patients' illnesses, *Time* did not consider that if a physician were to order surgery, or hospitalization, or send the patient home, without running adequate tests to validate his findings, he might *really* be guilty of poor practice of medicine and that his patients might then *legitimately* complain of rapid, impersonal, assembly-line treatment.

Less than a year later, in January, 1970, *Time*'s sister publication, *Fortune*, issued its own special report on "Our Ailing Medical System," calling for a discontinuation of fee-for-service medical practice (in which a patient pays a physician only for the care he receives, when he receives it).

The liberal *Washington Post*, in a 1970 editorial, embraced Senator Kennedy's proposal for national health insurance as "an idea so natural, so reasonable and so right that one wonders how the country could have floundered along for nearly two hundred years without it." Ignoring signs of increasing good health and long life in America, the *Post* stated, without any attempt at substantiation, that "the health record in this country is an appalling one for the bulk of its population."

CBS Television joined the campaign with two special one-hour programs in April, 1970, later turned into a book entitled *Don't Get Sick in America*, authored by CBS commentator Daniel Schorr.

There was no attempt at objectivity and balance in the CBS series. One network spokesman brushed off the bias in an interview with the *New York Daily News*: "If the program failed to accentuate the positive," he said, "that, in essence, is what journalism is all about." For months, representatives of American medicine fought for equal time to answer the attacks, but CBS refused.

Political and special interest publications joined the attack:

"National Health Plan Called Only Answer," reported the *AFL-CIO News*, in its issue of January 24, 1970.

In July of that year, *the body politic,* a publication of the left-wing Medical Committee for Human Rights, blamed doctors for pollution (because the AMA has not led the campaign for ecological improvement); for malnutrition (because it has not led the campaign for diet education); and for radioactivity. In its call for socialized medicine (including placing of social workers in charge of all clinics and hospitals) the magazine attacked the American Medical Association as "the dinosaur head of the medical-industrial complex."

Such was the nature of the attack in the media—an assault soon joined by newspapers and magazines in all sections of the country and all areas of public life. Women's magazines and *The New Repub-*

lic joined the chorus, and were joined in turn by such physician-oriented publications as *Medical Economics* ("Who says Americans abhor socialized medicine?") and *Medical World News* ("Birthday Bouquets for British Health Plan"), both of which are published by large non-medical publishing houses.

With leading Congressional liberals and labor spokesmen pounding furiously at the campaign's war drums, politicians and social activists from a wide variety of fields began to clamor about a health "crisis" and demand that "something be done"—usually in the form of national health insurance or some other program of greatly expanded government medicine.

—Civil rights leader Bayard Rustin urged Women's Liberation activists, who had called for equal employment opportunities in medicine, to make their demands "part of a larger demand for socialized medicine."

—Jerome Pollack, professor of economics at the Harvard Medical School, charged that "all or virtually all" Americans cannot afford to pay for their own medical care, and called for a system of universal (compulsory) health insurance, "now."

—Thomas J. Watson, Jr., chairman of the Board of Directors of International Business Machines Corp. (IBM), speaking at the Mayo Clinic in November, 1970, called the American system of medical care "decrepit" and concluded: "I believe we have only one choice before us that will work: some very new form of national health insurance."

In September, 1970, the Veterans Administration released a partial list of recent articles discussing national health insurance. There were nearly 130 entries, gleaned from such diverse publications as the *Wall Street Journal, Science News, New Republic, Business Week, Nation, The American Federationist, Business Horizons*, the *Washington Post, Science*, and a wide variety of medical and hospital publications.

As liberal politicians, mostly Democrats, began to respond in a race to enter their own national health insurance proposals, the Nixon administration, too, began to be moved by the relentless pressure. By mid-1970, the Department of Health, Education and Welfare had become the focal point of the administration's commitment. Near the end of the year, Dr. Vernon H. Wilson, HEW's third-ranking official, praised the Kennedy bill in a memorandum to Dr. Roger Egeberg, assistant HEW Secretary. Many of the bill's principles, Wilson said, "parallel proposals which we have been engaged in formulating . . ."

By the middle of 1971 the campaign for national health insurance had reached a crescendo. At least half a dozen major government health programs had been introduced into Congress.

Just six years ago, despite a 60-year campaign for national health insurance, the American public was still hesitant to involve government in non-military medical care. That debate seems to have ended; today, the nation argues over *which* plan shall be adopted.

The change has come about largely by default. Stung by the passage of Medicare and Medicaid, stunned by a massive propaganda campaign, large segments of the medical profession have come to believe that some form of national health insurance program is inevitable. The prophecy is self-fulfilling; by accepting the theory that government control is inevitable and acting accordingly, the profession may, indeed, prove it to be so.

Many in the medical profession—and on the Republican side of the aisles in Congress—have abandoned the battle against government medicine. The battle has become one for position only: "If *we* don't introduce a program, *they* will."

The result has been a plethora of health schemes. Those who limit their debate to "What Plan?" will have many to choose from (see Appendix II). Programs have been introduced by Republicans as well as Democrats; by "conservatives" as well as "liberals"; by the American Medical Association itself, as well as by its old foes, the AFL-CIO and the UAW. Most of the Democratic presidential aspirants have their names on bills as sponsors or co-sponsors, and President Nixon has introduced a plan of his own.

The reasons are varied: The AMA is following the position theory—let's do the controlling ourselves before *they* do it to us; the AFL-CIO and the UAW are continuing on a course of proposing radical social and economic change; the politicians—both Republican and Democrat—are responding to the propaganda efforts and political pressures in an attempt to guarantee election or re-election.

So far there are few signs of public arousal over the issue. Indeed, the well-publicized "public" cries for change seem to be coming entirely from a few politicians, social reformers, and journalists. But the drive, limited as it is, will have its effect. Though the news media may not be accurately reporting current public sentiment, it may well *create* the demands for change.

Already the results are beginning to show: For example, false comparisons of infant mortality statistics, which leave an impression of second-rate medical care in the U.S., have been widely circulated, and are now repeated in editorials and quoted in speeches as accepted fact. The public, bombarded with criticisms of "expensive" health care, has had its attention focused on rising costs in that area and the grumbling is beginning to pick up tempo. The critics fail to compare the increased costs in health care with increased costs in other fields—a study that would clearly identify politically created economic policies, and not the health care system, as the culprit.

It is such propaganda efforts that have frightened the medical profession into submission, and planted the seeds for an eventual public demand that "something be done." This is where the advocates of national health insurance come into the picture. The "something" that must be done, they say, is the creation of a new Federal medical system that will, according to its sponsors, increase the quality of medical care and reduce its costs.

The facts, of course, are quite different, as I will attempt to demonstrate. But the campaign may work. Indeed, it now appears that unless a counter-effort develops rapidly, the United States may soon replace the familiar family physician with a new and impersonal system of mass medical care under Federal control.

Labor's long campaign appears to be paying off.

3. The American Murder Association

Underlying the campaign for national health insurance are three European philosophical concepts that have never been well accepted in the United States: socialistic egalitarianism (all goods and all wealth should be redistributed by the state to each person according to his need); Hegelian statism (man exists to serve the needs of the state); and an arrogant royalist or baronial elitism, by means of which some presume the right to regulate others.

Obviously, promoters of government medical programs would face an enormous task in trying to sell socialism to a people who have seen their nation grow great and its individuals prosper as a result of private enterprise incentives. Similarly, they would have a difficult chore in trying to sell the statist concept of a benevolent and omnipotent government to a people who have repeatedly opted for freedom when the choices were clear before them. But the debate does not take place behind such awesome terms as egalitarianism and Hegelian statism. Philosophy is seldom discussed and the argument is skillfully directed away from such clear-cut choices as (a) private enterprise or (b) government regulation.

Instead the campaign moves behind catch phrases and slogans ranging from the shrill cry of the far left that the American Medical Association is really "the American Murder Association" to a more moderate insistence that America is in the midst of a national health "crisis" for which *something* must be done.

In July, 1969, left-wing students marched on the American Medical Association's annual convention in New York City, shouting "Hip, Hip, Hippocrates! Up with service, down with fees." When the AMA offered the demonstrators time at the speaker's platform, Richard Kunnes, a young New Yorker who had refused to stand for the national anthem, stormed to the rostrum and accused the AMA of being an organization of "criminals," and a "murder association" responsible for "the needless deaths of countless millions of people."

The charges were repeated in *the body politic,* the "journal" of the far-left Medical Committee for Human Rights. MCHR is ostensibly a legitimate medical organization. Its principal spokesman, Dr. Quentin Young, has no difficulty in finding outlets to voice his views in the media; MCHR statements are duly reported as significant utterances in the medical-social world. Press coverage usually fails to identify either Dr. Young or MCHR other than as representative of a dissident group of liberal physicians, concerned with the alleged failings of American medicine.

The MCHR journal more clearly reveals the true nature of this organization, which has initiated much of the attack on American medicine. On page one of the issue for July/August, 1970, a cartoon shows an AMA superman towering over a squirming mass of living skeletons, resembling the survivors of Dachau. On page two, an article by Quentin Young is illustrated with a drawing of a Chicago policeman, his pants open and his penis showing, holding up the dress of a tearful Miss Liberty, whose underdrawers are open. On the next page, a cartoon pictures a host of grotesquely caricatured physicians, one of whom is shouting, ". . . To us, there are no poor!"

In the accompanying article, Young accuses the AMA of "inextricable ties to the military industrial predators," and sums up the theme of the 1970 anti-AMA demonstrations that received prominent nationwide news coverage:

"End racism in the health care delivery system.
"End oppression of women by and in the system.
"End war-collaboration by the health industry.
"Socialize the health care system."

In the same issue, *the body politic* repeated Kunnes' 1969 charges in New York. In an article entitled "American Murder Association," Kunnes alleges that the AMA is a "death profession." The article is illustrated with a skeleton AMA clutching a fistful of money, a ghoulish Uncle Sam, and a bloated "capitalist" complete with top hat and a dollar sign on his tie.

In a portion of the article that clearly links the MCHR attack on American medicine with radical assaults on the United States in general, Kunnes rails against "expansionistic and imperialistic" medical centers, and an "exploitative capitalistic system," which he says must be "crushed." Later the magazine presents a cartoon of Hitler, comparing American "atrocities" to those of Nazi Germany. Although convinced that Americans are not yet up to his own standards, the cartoon Hitler concludes, "They're learning." And on page 30, Eli C. Messinger, national chairman of MCHR, writes of the committee's "fellowship" with the violent Black Panthers.

Obviously the Medical Committee for Human Rights is not the only critic of American medical care. Yet it is essential that the public learn the true story of MCHR and its ultra-leftist ties, for the committee has been a prime instigator of the assault on American medicine and its criticisms have been widely reported as those of a respectable medical society. Regularly since 1965, MCHR has been picketing AMA meetings, receiving widespread news coverage of its charges of racism, second-rate medical care, high fees and a failing medical system. Many of the cries initiated by the MCHR have found their way into more respectable circles, where they have been repeated with an air of certainty and again spread through the press to the public.

For example, the *National Observer*, in a feature article in its issue for July 21, 1969, identified Kunnes and his co-demonstrators merely as "200 or so young people." James G. Driscoll, author of the *National Observer* article, implied that the group's "unhappiness"—and a "growing" leftist movement in the medical field—stemmed innocently from doctor shortages, medical care costs and other "widespread concerns about health care." The *Observer* devoted five paragraphs to publicizing Kunnes' charges, without revealing the nature of the Medical Committee for Human Rights as a part of the widespread radical assault on the entire American system of individual freedoms.

The sloganeering, however, has not been limited to the MCHR radicals. Other less radical voices cry as shrilly about a so-called "massive health crisis."

"Today, almost everyone is talking about the crisis in health care," William Schnitzler, secretary-treasurer of the AFL-CIO, told a pharmaceutical conference at Rutgers in 1969.

The national health insurance program introduced by Senator Edward Kennedy "will provide . . . solutions to the health care crisis," Leonard Woodcock, president of the United Auto Workers, said when he assumed chairmanship of the Committee for National Health Insurance in June, 1970.

"The deepening health care crisis . . . is a matter of grave concern," Roger Egeberg, Assistant Secretary of the Department of Health, Education and Welfare, told business leaders at a Harvard Club meeting in January, 1970.

And so it has gone. Even President Nixon, not wishing to be outdone, has publicly stated that America is in the midst of a "massive health crisis."

Such slogans, whether the cry of campus radicals or the President of the United States, have one common thrust: to pave the way for some form of new system by convincing the American public that its health care is inadequate, unavailable and inordinately costly.

Essentially, the attack has followed these lines:

1.   There is a crisis in medical treatment, evidenced primarily by a high rate of infant mortality.

2.   Medical and health care bills are outrageously high and many Americans can no longer afford to pay for medical treatment.

3.   There is a critical doctor shortage and a serious maldistribution of those doctors who are available.

4.   There is no efficient system for delivery of health care services in the United States.

5.   Private doctors, free to make whatever they can, are frequently dishonest at a high cost to the individual patient and to the taxpayer.

Among the specific charges:

—A baby born in the United States has less chance of surviving the first month of life than do infants in fourteen countries—evidence that the United States is a second-rate country in providing health care.

—In some areas (for example, the Watts section of Los Angeles and parts of Boston), there is only one physician for every 4–5,000 residents.

—Health care costs are rising faster than the cost of other goods and services. The nation's health care bill has risen to $70 billion a year—three times the health expenditures a decade ago.

Senator Kennedy, in his introduction to Daniel Schorr's book *Don't Get Sick in America,* calls for a health "revolution"—a revolution that may well come if Americans conclude that the charges leveled against the free-enterprise medical system are true.

In the following chapters, we shall review these major criticisms one at a time, and see what merit, if any, they possess.

PART TWO

THE "CRISIS"

4. The Health Care "Crisis"

"For the great majority of Americans, the health care crisis is not a TV show or a presidential address; it is an on-going crisis of survival."

With those words, Barbara and John Ehrenreich, co-authors of an anti-free enterprise polemic entitled *The American Health Empire*, continued the massive—and almost unquestioned—campaign to link the words "health" and "crisis" as inextricably as American League baseball teams, Broadway playgoers and Southerners once linked the words "Damn" and "Yankee."

"For the great majority of Americans," say the Ehrenreichs, the matter of health care has become a *"crisis of survival."* The statement is ridiculous on its face and easily disproved on a purely empirical basis. The reader need only take a few moments to consider his own case, that of his friends and relatives, and that of his fellow workers, to determine whether a *great majority* are indeed faced with a *crisis of survival* because of inability to obtain decent medical care. Pressed, the makers of the crisis theory will usually back down to a more moderate position: "large numbers of persons in the 'ghettos' and in rural areas are unable to afford good medical care, or to find doctors to provide it" (a thesis that I hope to disprove with this and succeeding chapters).

But those who advocate a national medical revolution—govern-

ment insurance for *everybody*—will have a difficult time selling such
a program on the basis of providing for the needs of that small
percentage of Americans who do not have private health insurance.
(More than eight out of ten Americans *are* insured privately.)
Therefore, it becomes essential to avoid a debate on the questions:
how many Americans do not have access to health care; how many
cannot afford it; how many are not privately insured; how many
have medical bills that create a serious threat to financial security?
To discuss these questions, after all, leaves the arena free for the
introduction of such facts as (a) the United States has one of the
world's highest per capita physician populations; (b) the average
middle-income American spends only seven percent of his annual
expenditures on goods and services for medical insurance and
medical care, and (c) all Americans—all ages and all races—are
enjoying a health care "boom," producing longer life and sturdier
bodies. (These facts will all be documented in the following pages.)

Thus the attempt to hide the campaign behind cliches and slogans. "We are the richest and most powerful country on earth,"
says Alex Gerber, author of *The Gerber Report,* a book on the
"shocking state of American medical care." So, "Why are we not
the healthiest?"

Gerber, too, was repeating a popular catch phrase: "Why are we
not the healthiest?" The "proof" of that statement is usually found
to rest primarily on a United Nations comparison of infant mortality rates—a comparison that is clearly invalid (and stated to be so
in the UN report), and that totally ignores a whole series of charts
in the same report that lead to a totally different conclusion.

The "damnyankee" sloganeering—the "healthcrisis" theme—is
intentional. Though there is no health crisis—not even a serious
health problem—in the United States, the advocates of national
health insurance know that a charge that is repeated often enough,
by enough people, and spread by means of the public media into
every home over a long period of time, will eventually come to be
accepted as true, even though those who use the word cannot
substantiate their statements and usually do not even try.

One must use care in his choice of words, for words have precise
meanings. The word "crisis," for example, means (according to
Webster's dictionary) either (a) the turning point in an acute disease or fever; (b) a paroxysmal attack of distress or disordered

function; (c) a radical change of status; (d) a decisive moment; or (e) an unstable or crucial time.

Only from the standpoint of definition (d)—"a decisive moment"—can there be said to exist a "crisis" in medicine. But *that* crisis is political and philosophical, not medical, in its nature. In no regard can it be said that there exists a "crisis" in health care. Medical care in this country is not in distress; there has been no instability and no radical change (indeed, the advocates of national health insurance have been crying that medical care was inadequate and its cost exorbitant for at least 40 years). Instead, medical care progresses at a wondrous rate, sometimes spectacularly, to provide better health and longer life for each succeeding generation.

The word "crisis" has a specific meaning, like other words, and is not to be bandied about in any fashion that may please its user; yet, that is just what is being done today by those who, with great irresponsibility, speak of a health "crisis" in the United States. The misuse is not only intentional; it is devious. Those who use the phrase to promote government medicine do so knowing that the public will attach to the word its *true* meaning, and thus assume that the user does know of an *actual* "crisis"—a situation that must be met with drastic action somehow to save the day.

Let us examine that "crisis."

One valid manner of measuring the progressive improvement in medical care is a comparison between life expectancies past and present.

Much of the world's past greatness has been snuffed out by early death. For example, Robert Burns died at 37; Kafka at 41; Van Dyck at 42; Mozart at 35. Of the three famous Bronte sisters, only one lived beyond her 20's. Chekhov was dead, of consumption, at the age of 44, and John Keats at the age of 26.

Consumption—tuberculosis—has now been practically wiped out as a potential killer. If Chekhov and Keats had lived in the United States of today, they might have produced masterpieces of literature for far longer than a meager 44 and 26 years.

The tragic early deaths of Keats and Chekhov, of Mozart and Burns and the Brontes, were typical of the age. Just 100 years ago, the average American could expect to die before his 42nd birthday.

Dr. Wesley W. Hall, president of the American Medical Association, recently wrote, "We can still do only one thing: exercise some influence upon the time and cause of death." By that standard, modern health care performs miracles unthought of when this century began.

Diseases that killed hundreds of thousands in the past have been virtually wiped out of existence. Tuberculosis and polio are prominent examples. The death rate from uterine cancer has been cut in half in the last 30 years. Open-heart surgery has become almost commonplace and saves many lives each year.

Most middle-aged Americans—even many still fairly young ones —can remember the sad sight of children walking painfully in stiff metal braces as a result of the crippling effects of polio—the same illness that turned Franklin D. Roosevelt, a robust young man, into a wheelchair invalid. Many can still remember the sight of signs nailed to the front doors of houses, warning visitors to stay away for fear of catching the "whooping cough" that lurked inside. Many can remember the formaldehyde-soaked bedsheets isolating the suffering victims of scarlet fever, and the ritual burning of the patient's bed clothing, pajamas, towels—anything that had touched the victim of the disease.

Those days are gone forever. Today, reports of whooping cough or scarlet fever in a hospital would bring interns rushing to study the disease—an illness they might never come across again in their years of practice.

Statistics clearly reveal the falsehood of charges that America is in the midst of a medical-care "crisis."

—Life expectancy at birth has increased from 41 years in 1850, and only 49 years in 1900, to more than 70 years today.

—In 1850, a fourth of the newborn died before age five; in 1900, a fourth of the newborn died before age 25; today, only a fourth of the newborn will fail to reach age 62. In fact, according to the *New York Times' Encyclopedic Almanac* for 1970, half of today's newborn are likely to live at least 74 years.

Many of the diseases and illnesses that afflict all ages have been subdued, in part, by the advances of modern medical care. Americans at every age—even into their 70s—can expect still more life ahead of them than an American of the same age at the turn of the century.

Figures released in the 1971 *Statistical Abstract of the U.S.* lead to similar conclusions:

—The life expectancy at birth for all Americans, white and Negro, in 1920 was 54.1 years. By 1930 the life expectancy had increased to 59.7 years; by 1940 it was nearly 63 years. Today it is 70.5 years (67.0 for males and 74.2 for females).

—Of every 1,000 white male Americans at age 20 in 1921, 4.27 died before their 21st birthday; today the mortality rate at age 20 has been reduced to 1.77. For females, the rate has dropped from 4.33 to 0.61.

—The mortality rate for males at age 40 has dropped from 7.50 per 1,000 in 1900 to 3.37 today; for females, the rate has dropped from 6.76 to 1.93.

—At age 65, the mortality rate has dropped from 34.99 to 33.61 for males, *and from 31.68 to 16.17 for females!*

Life expectancy has increased at every stage of life:

—In 1921, the average white male at age 20 could expect to live another 45.6 years; today he can look forward to another 50.2 years. The average white female at age 20 in 1921 had approximately 46.5 years left to live; today she has another 56.9 years.

—In 1921, the average white male at age 40 could expect to live another 29.86 years, and the female could expect another 30.94 years. Today the male can expect an additional 31.8 years, and the female another 37.8 years.

—In 1921, the average white male at age 65 could expect to live another 12.21 years and the female 12.75 years; today, the male can expect approximately 13 more years, and the female can expect approximately 16.5 more years, an increase of nearly four years.

There are other indicators, too:

—In 1921, fewer than 85,000 out of every 100,000 white males lived to the age of 20; today the figure is in excess of 96,000 out of every 100,000.

—In 1921, only 75,733 of every 100,000 white males lived to the age of 40; today the figure is 92,583. (Note the very slight drop between the number who reach age 20 and the number who live to age 40.)

—In 1921, only 50,663 of every 100,000 white males lived to be 65; in 1941, the figure was up to 58,305; in 1951, up to 63,541; today, it is nearly 66,000.

—In 1921, only 54,229 of every 100,000 white females lived to

the age of 65; today, that figure is up to 81,486 of every 100,000
—*an increase of a full 50 percent!*

Clearly there is no longevity crisis among the white population
of America. Critics of the free enterprise medical system, however,
claim that there is a wide disparity between the quality of medical
care available to the rich and the poor; the white and the black. Let
us consider, then, whether or not there is a longevity "crisis"
among the Negro population in America.

The figures for black Americans are lower in most categories
than they are for whites—a fact largely attributable to non-medical
factors, such as improper diet, inadequate income, employment at
hard labor and lower quality housing. Yet the statistics reveal that
even among black Americans there is, rather than a "crisis," significant progress in terms of maintained health and sustained life.

For example:

—In 1920, the average Negro male had a life expectancy at birth
of 45.5 years; today, his average life expectancy is 61.1 years.

—In 1920, the average Negro female had a life expectancy at
birth of 45.2 years; today, her average life expectancy is 68.2 years.

—The "gap" between the life expectancies of the white and
black populations has narrowed from nearly 10 years in 1920 (45.3
and 54.9) to less than seven years today (64.6 versus 71.3).

—In 1921, more than 10 percent of all Negro babies died at
birth; today, the rate is down to less than four percent.

—In 1921, 14.59 of every 100,000 black Americans who
reached the age of 40 died before their 41st birthday; today, that
rate is down to 8.68 of every 100,000.

—In 1921, the average Negro American who lived to age 65
could expect another 12.07 years of life (male) or another 12.41
years (female). Today, the expectancy at age 65 is 12.7 years (male)
and 15.8 years (female).

—In 1921, only 79,057 out of every 100,000 Negro males lived
to the age of 20; today, nearly 94,000 live 20 years.

—In 1921, only 61,353 of every 100,000 Negro males (and only
61,130 of the Negro females) lived to age 40. Today, 85,013 of
every 100,000 males and more than 90,000 of every 100,000
females live to age 40.

—In 1921, only 34,042 of every 100,000 Negro males reached
age 65; today, the figure is 50,180.

—In 1921, only 31,044 of every 100,000 Negro females reached age 65; today, the figure is 64,255—*more than twice as many!*

There is no question that the average American Negro—for many reasons—has a shorter life expectancy than the average white American. In some age groups, there has been no progress at all: for example, the mortality rate among Negro males at age 65 has actually increased since 1921. Similarly, from age 40 on, the longevity increases for Negro males have been relatively small.

Yet it is equally clear that the trend has been toward improvement, rather than deterioration of medical care. Overall life expectancy for Negroes has increased dramatically during this century, as it has for whites. The percentage of Negroes living to ages 20, 40 and 65 has also increased sharply. The life-expectancy gap between whites and blacks has been gradually reduced.

In these terms, there is no more of a medical or health care "crisis" for blacks than for white Americans.

For a medical "crisis" to exist only for the black community would imply that there is a marked difference in the care available to the white and black American—or, as it is stated by advocates of national health insurance, between the rich and the poor. If that were the case, there would be substantial differences between the races in life expectancy at all stages of life, particularly in the later years, when health depends more and more upon medical care. The facts reveal just the opposite. From age 40 on, the difference in life expectancy between white males and Negro males is very slight. At age 40, the difference is 3.5 years; at age 47 it is down to 2.5 years; at age 53 it is down to 1.7 years. The average white American male at age 55 can look forward to another 19.5 years of life; the average black American male at the same age can expect another 18 years of life—1.5 years difference.

The gap narrows still more at age 60, when members of both races become increasingly dependent upon medical care—and when retirement narrows the other, non-medical, differences between the living standards of the races. At age 60, the average white American male can expect another 16.1 years of life; the average Negro male 15.3 years. At age 65, the average white male can expect another 13 years of life; the average Negro male another 12.7 years—or almost the same life expectancy, at a time when that expectancy is very much dependent upon the quality of health services.

In fact, using available statistics, it could well be argued that the current medical system favors black Americans; for at a time when dependence on that system is greatest—age 67 and older—the Negro has a *greater* expectancy of continued life than does the white of the same age.

Obviously it would be fallacious to attempt to deduce from such official government statistics any claim that the health of Negro Americans is as good, generally, as that of the white population. There *is* a gap. But the figures do indicate two things clearly: (1) There is no health "crisis" in terms of longevity for either whites or blacks. The quality of care is not deteriorating; it is improving rapidly. (2) Differences between the life expectancies of whites and blacks do not indicate failings of the medical system, per se, but rather point up the health drain of primarily non-medical factors inherent in different living standards, different diets, etc.

Similarly, the existence of a health "crisis" is belied by a study of the causes of death between 1950 and 1967 (the latest year for which figures are available). Although there are some diseases in which medicine has made little progress, if any (for example, the malignancy death rate has increased 1.7 percent), there are other areas in which the progress has been quite significant:

—In 1950, 22.5 of every 100,000 Americans died of tuberculosis; today the rate is down to 3.5.

—In 1950, five of every 100,000 Americans died of syphilis, compared to 1.2 today (at a time when medical reports reveal a major increase in the incidence of venereal diseases).

—In 1950, 1.3 of every 100,000 Americans died of acute poliomyelitis; in 1967, there were only 16 polio deaths in the entire nation.

—The death rate from hypertensive heart disease has been reduced from 56.5 per 100,000 in 1950, to 25.3 in 1967.

There have also been marked decreases in the *incidence* of many diseases. The following figures are taken from the *Statistical Abstract of the U.S.* (1971), table 107, page 78:

—More than 18,600 cases of diphtheria were reported in the United States in 1945; by 1968, the figure was down to 260.

—The number of reported cases of malaria was reduced from 62,763 in 1945 to 2,317 in 1968.

—The number of reported cases of measles was reduced from

146,013 in 1945 to 22,231 in 1968.

—The number of meningococcal infections fell from 8,208 to 2,623 during that period.

—The number of cases of whooping cough fell from 133,792 to 4,810.

—The number of cases of acute poliomyelitis fell from 13,625 to only 53.

—Reported cases of typhoid fever fell from 4,211 to 395.

The report *also* includes diseases that have been reported in *increased* frequency, possibly because of new reporting procedures, possibly because of actual increased incidence. It is not my intention to interpret these figures nor to maintain that medicine has *conquered* disease; it *has* made *some* progress against *some* diseases; it *has* made *wondrous* progress against others.

Neither is it my intention to claim that all of the credit for this progress goes to the individual practicing physician. The decrease of incidence, like the decrease in mortality from many of these diseases, is not so much attributable to better care in the physician's office as to

(1) medical *scientists*—researchers—who have produced their discoveries in a variety of ways (privately with use of private funds, privately with Federal funds, or in Federal research centers with Federal funds);

(2) free enterprise pharmaceutical manufacturers, who continue to develop and produce high-quality, lifesaving drug products and make them available to the nation's physicians;

(3) widespread immunization programs, sponsored either by private organizations (for example, county medical societies) or local governments.

It is not my desire to claim that all progress is due to the efforts of private practitioners. It *is* my desire, however, to show conclusively that there is no medical crisis in the United States. These figures, and the tables and charts showing great increases in longevity and decreases in disease mortality, as well as figures showing a reduction in the incidence of a number of formerly fatal diseases, show conclusively that (a) health care today is good, and (b) that it is continually getting better.

At any rate, it seems clear that, so far as progress against specific diseases is concerned, there is no medical *crisis* in the United States.

There is yet another indicator of significance. One might expect that in a nation suffering a "crisis" in health care, and in which medical care is not available to large segments of the public, the population would be stunted in growth and small in frame. Just the opposite is true in the United States. "Vociferous critics of U.S. medicine, who recite infant mortality statistics as proof health care here is the worst in the western world, may be called on in the future to explain why, if this is so, Americans are fast becoming the biggest people on earth," *Medical News Report* said recently.

The report referred to a recent government study, released by the U.S. Department of Health, Education and Welfare, which revealed that American children between ages 6 and 11 are taller and heavier, on the average, than in any other national population. According to the HEW study, American children have increased in height by at least half an inch each decade for the past 90 years, and have increased in weight by 15 to 30 percent. The average eight-year-old boy of today, said the report, is almost 4.5 inches taller and up to 19 pounds heavier than the eight-year-old boy of 1880.

Adults are correspondingly taller and heavier, the report revealed.

Dr. Peter V. Hamill, chief medical advisor for the study, observed: "Generally speaking, it is an index of good national health when the population is tall and weighs enough." He credited nutrition, exercise—and the medical advances of the past century that have greatly reduced the harmful effects of many childhood diseases and infections.

Nutrition, of course, *is* a major factor in the increased size of the average American, as it is a factor in the increased length of life. Yet it seems irrefutably clear that nutrition improvements or not, if Americans were receiving a low grade of medical care, the health of Americans would be much lower and, conversely, if Americans are generally fit, as seems to be the case, that a good part of that fitness is due to the health maintenance provided by American physicians and the medical system in this country.

The most often repeated criticism of American medical care (aside from those of "high cost" and the "doctor shortage," both of which will be discussed in later chapters) is the claim that the United States ranks 11th or worse among world nations in *infant mortality.* The implication is twofold: first, that the United States has a *crisis* in terms of infant mortality; second, that health care in the United States is inferior to that in other countries. To examine the validity of these implications, we must first study the current rate of infant mortality in the United States, as contrasted with rates in earlier years (the "crisis" argument), and then look into the accuracy of the contention that the cited statistics prove that American health care is inferior to that available in other countries (the "comparison" argument.)

A. The "Crisis" Argument

In 1970, the infant mortality rate in the United States reached an all-time low of 19.8 deaths per 1,000 live births—a decrease of 4.3 percent from the 1969 rate of 20.7. In fact, the latest reduction in the infant mortality rate is part of a consistent trend. At the beginning of this century, *124.5* of every 1,000 infants died within the first year of life. By 1940, the rate was down to 47 per 1,000.

Those who cry "crisis" frequently maintain that the improvement in mortality rates was registered in the early years of the century, and that American medicine has been stagnant since. The facts are just the opposite. It is true, of course, that once a certain point is reached, the rate of improvement must slow. Given the many factors involved in an infant death, it is unlikely that the infant mortality rate wil' ever approach zero—and it is likely that unless it does, those who criticize in order to create change will continue to find fault. But the rate *does* continue to improve. Between 1940 and 1945 the rate dropped nearly nine points—to 38.3 infant deaths per 1,000. By 1950 it had dropped to 29.2. By 1960 it was down to 26 per 1,000.

Despite the claims of those who would destroy the system, the truth is simply that impi ovement continues at a significant rate. In fact, the nation's infant mortality rate improved by a full 24 percent in the last decade from 26 per 1,000 in 1960 to 19.8 in 1970. The current rate (19.8) is slightly more than *half* the 1945 infant death rate.

The infant mortality rate represents the number of infants who die within less than one year after birth. Statistics reveal marked improvements also in the fetal death rate (stillbirths) and the neonatal death rate (fetus deaths within 28 days of conception). The fetal death rate decreased from 23.9 in 1945 to 15.6 in 1967. The neonatal death rate decreased from 28.8 in 1940 to 20.5 in 1950, 18.7 in 1960, and 15.8 in 1968.

Perhaps the most signicant sign of advancement in medical care during the past three decades has been in the prevention of maternal deaths (deaths during delivery). Only 30 years ago, in 1940, 376 of every 100,000 births resulted in the death of the mother. Today that figure has been reduced to a low 28 per 100,000 (1967 figures).

Again, though the rates for Negro Americans are not quite as good as those for whites, there has been a significant improvement in all four categories for blacks as well.

The infant mortality rate for Negroes was 73.8 per 1,000 in 1940 —more than 30 points higher than that for whites (43.2). By 1970 the Negro infant mortality rate was down to 35.9—less than half what it had been only three decades earlier, and only 16 points higher than that for whites (19.7). Not only had the death rate been cut in half, so had the gap between whites and blacks.

What is more, the improvement trend has been consistent. In 1940, the Negro infant mortality rate was 73.8; in 1950, it was 44.5; in 1960, it was 43.2; in 1970, 32.5.

The same has been true of the fetal death rate. In 1945, 42 of every 1,000 Negro fetuses were stillborn; today the rate is down to 25.8. And similarly in the neonatal death rate. In 1940, 39.7 of every 1,000 Negro fetuses died in the womb; in 1967, the figure was down to 23.8.

The maternal death rate among Negro women remains considerably higher than that for white women, but here, too, there has been remarkable improvement. In 1940, 773.5 of every 100,000 Negro mothers died during delivery; in 1967, that rate was down to 69.5 of every 100,000, less than 10 percent of the rate only 30 years earlier.

Clearly, the infant mortality criticism is false insofar as it leads to the conclusion that there is an infant mortality "crisis" in the United States. In truth, American medicine has made remarkable improvement in the prevention of infant mortality, fetal mortality, neonatal mortality and maternal mortality in this century—with much of the progress occuring during the last 30 years.

B. The Comparison Argument

Of the many criticisms leveled at the American medical system, none is repeated more often, nor with more damaging effect, than the charge that infant mortality rates in the United States are much higher than those in other nations—nations with national health programs, of course.

Those who make such claims frequently are unable to cite the source of their information. The charge has been so often repeated, so widely disseminated through speeches and original articles, and so widely reported by the news media, that it is often accepted as fact and repeated uncritically at all levels of communication. It is important, however, to know the source of such information, and the validity (or lack of it) claimed for the information by its originator.

The figures are usually selected from a report published by the World Health Organization, which lists nine nations with lower infant mortality rates than that of the United States, or from a monograph published by the U.S. Public Health Service, which lists 13 nations with lower infant death rates.

Both lists, however, contain the same flaws. They *are* accurate, presumably, in terms of reporting a nation's infant death rate according to the criteria followed in that nation; for various reasons, they are *not* suitable for purposes of comparison—a fact admitted by both the UN and the Public Health Service, but conveniently overlooked by those who compare for political purposes.

In effect, comparing the infant mortality rates of different nations is much like comparing apples and oranges. If one determines optimum desirability from the standards set by apple growers—for example, smoothness of skin, redness of color, whiteness of interior —one can easily conclude that the apple is a superior fruit. Obviously, the standards are *not* the same, and comparisons are meaningless.

So it is with international comparisons of infant mortality statistics. Here are some of the ways in which the apples differ from the oranges.

1.   Critics frequently compare 1968 infant mortality figures for the United States (20.8) and Sweden (12.9). The implication, of course, is that the U.S. should adopt the Swedish system of

socialized medicine. There are, however, *important differences between the two countries and their people.* Among them:

(a) The United States has a population of more than 200 million people; Sweden has a population of about 8 million—or slightly *more* than the state of New Jersey and slightly *less* than the state of Michigan.

(b) The United States is more nearly a continent than a nation in size, covering 3.6 million square miles (about the same size as all of Europe, and thus covering many different climates). Sweden covers 175,000 square miles (about the size of the state of California).

(c) The U.S. has an extremely *heterogeneous* population, made up of representatives of all races and ethnic groups, and widely diverse social and cultural backgrounds. The population of Sweden, on the other hand is relatively *homogeneous.*

Indeed, comparisons between infant mortality rates for *white Americans only,* on the one hand, and the predominantly white populations of a *similar area* in northwestern Europe (including 12 countries), produces a much different result: an infant mortality rate of 20.6 for the U.S. (1965–67) compared with a rate of 20.3 for the European countries. In other words, when comparing apples with apples, the rates are almost identical.

Those who complain about infant mortality rates in the U.S. point out that the *rate* for northwestern Europe has improved 35 percent since 1955–57, compared with an improvement of only 12 percent for the white U.S. population. This is merely an example of European medical care *catching up;* in the period 1955–57, the infant mortality rate in northwest Europe was 31.2 deaths per 1,000 live births, compared with 23.4 among white Americans.

It is interesting to note that those who cite infant mortality comparisons do so very selectively. For example, one seldom hears the U.S. figures compared to those in South America or in the Soviet Union. In 1970, there were 19.8 infant deaths in the U.S. for every 1,000 live births. There were 26 infant deaths per 1,000 live births in the Soviet Union, and from 46 (Venezuela) to 108 (Chile) in South America.

If one compares selectively, rather than using similar populations and areas, it is possible to produce almost any sort of desired result

—as the advocates of national health insurance have done.

For example, it is true that the U.S. cannot match the low infant mortality rates in the homogeneous Scandinavian countries of Norway, Sweden, and Denmark. On the other hand, the infant mortality rate for whites in the U.S. is generally lower than the rate for Germany (which has a national health program), and about the same as the rate for France (which has a national health program). Similarly, the infant mortality rate for whites in the Middle Atlantic states is similar to the combined rate for Great Britain and Ireland; the rate in New Jersey is about the same as in England and Wales; the rate in Utah has been as low as those in Denmark or Switzerland.

The comparison between the U.S. and northwestern Europe includes the European nations of Sweden, Norway, Denmark, Finland, the Netherlands, Switzerland, England, Wales, Scotland, Ireland, Belgium, France and West Germany. If one were to compare all of the U.S. and *all* of Europe—including Italy, Spain and Portugal—the infant mortality rate for the U.S. would be considerably lower (20.6 white, 23.6 total for the U.S.; 26.2 for Europe).

It might be helpful at this point to consider the reasons why the infant mortality rate for black Americans is higher than that for whites. Longevity statistics reported earlier in this chapter—particularly those relating to years of expected additional life past the age of 60, when reliance on medical care is increased—suggest that the "fault" lies not in the system of medical treatment, but in other factors. There has been evidence cited to indicate that these differences are due primarily to certain sociological factors, including the past history of racial discrimination that has caused many Negroes to work in less desirable jobs, earn less pay, and consequently have a less favorable standard of living than that of white Americans. There is some evidence to substantiate this theory in a report in the *Bulletin* of the Greenville County (S.C.) Medical Society, which stated that the infant mortality rate among non-whites in California, where the non-white income level is comparatively high, is only slightly higher than the white infant mortality rate in the state of West Virginia, where incomes are relatively low.

Among the other apple and orange discrepancies that invalidate international comparisons of infant mortality rates:

2.   In some countries, such as Sweden, birth reports are not

required until five years after the event. In others, the report of birth is the responsibility of the parents. In many European nations, including the Netherlands and the Soviet Union, deliveries are frequently performed by a midwife. In all of these cases, there is an obvious likelihood that many births will go unreported.

In the United States, on the other hand, almost all births are by physician (3,462,000 by physician; 39,000 by midwife), and almost all are in a hospital (3,449,000 in hospital; 52,000 not in hospital). In the U.S., physicians are required to certify all deaths.

It seems clear that infant mortality rates in other nations are certain to look better as a result of the fact that almost all U.S. infant deaths are reported, while many infant deaths in other nations may not be reported.

3.   In nations with liberalized abortion laws, many impaired fetuses may be aborted—and thus not recorded either as births or infant deaths. In the United States, deformed fetuses go to term, are delivered, and frequently die, thus being included as infant deaths.

4.   Different nations have vastly different criteria for determining existence of a live birth. In some countries, a live birth is any fetus delivered 20 weeks or more after conception; in others, any fetus delivered after 28 weeks; in others, any fetus that weighs at least 1,000 grams (2.2 pounds) at birth; in others, any that breathes; in others, any that exhibits voluntary muscle movement.

It is obviously impossible to compare a 27-week fetus delivered in one nation with a 1,000-gram fetus delivered in another. Yet that is what is done by those who compare international infant mortality statistics. Statistical methods are not comparable *within* the United States (the official U.S. figure is an average of figures reported by various states, each using its own laws and requirements); they are even less comparable when considering a 350-gram (0.75 pound) live birth in Kansas with a 900-gram fetus delivered in another nation and not recorded as a live birth or subsequent infant death.

As a further example, 39 states in the U.S. call the death of any infant delivered 20 weeks after conception a neonatal death; in the Netherlands ("ranked" second in the WHO table) and Norway (third), a fetus that dies at any time prior to the *28th* week after conception is not counted in mortality tables.

Dr. John R. Schenken, of the University of Nebraska, has

pointed out that "in countries where the average individual stature is smaller than in the United States, the viable infant is likewise smaller. If the United States' weight requirements are applied in those countries, the infant mortality rates would naturally be much lower than in the United States."

5.   The United States has a higher proportion of births to mothers under age 20. According to the report by the Greenville County Medical Society, 17.2 percent of all U.S. births in 1967 were to mothers in their teens (15 percent among whites, 27.9 percent among non-whites). This rate compares to 12.1 percent in Sweden, 11.6 percent in Denmark, 10.4 percent in Finland "and even smaller proportions in other European countries" (using 1965 figures).

"Young mothers have more premature births," the report said, "and prematurely born infants (or infants with low birth weight) account for two-thirds of the deaths among the newborn."

The *comparison* argument is obviously invalid. The statistics reported for the various nations included in the WHO and PHS reports are *not comparable*. What is more, both reports say as much.

The United Nations disclaims comparison reliability in its *Demographic Yearbook for 1968* (page 28):

"Limitations: Infant death statistics are subject to all the limitations of vital statistics in general and of death and live birth statistics in particular.

"Perhaps the most important and widespread limitation on comparability results from compiling statistics of infant deaths and live births by date of registration rather than date of occurrence of the events. Where these procedures obtain, a large increase, for whatever reason, in the number of live births registered in any one year, may introduce sizable errors into the infant mortality rates, especially since deaths tend to be more promptly reported than births.

"If the delay in registration remains nearly constant and is approximately the same for births and deaths, the rates are not affected to any appreciable degree. But if—*as is the case in many countries*—a large proportion of the births are not registered until many years after occurrence, then infant mortality rates obtained by relating deaths for any one year to births which occurred over a period of years *have little validity*" (emphasis added).

The Public Health Service Monograph contains a similar disclaimer about the validity of comparing "disconnected studies with varying study designs."

"Although a few comparisons may be possible fortuitously," the report said, "they lack the assurance which is to be derived from a well-designed study planned to give answers to specific questions."

These disclaimers are in the reports from which the critics of free enterprise medicine draw the "comparisons" that they use to indict American medical care. To compare the incomparable—to compare apples and oranges—and to hide the disclaimers published by the originating sources is dishonest and deceitful. Nowhere do the advocates of government medical controls more clearly show their willingness to distort and mislead in an attempt to fool the public into accepting their schemes.

Clearly the infant mortality comparisons are deceitful. But, surprisingly (considering the prominence given to such charges), they are also relatively meaningless as a basis for judging the efficacy of a nation's health system.

For one thing, infant mortality is more nearly a social problem than a medical problem: malnutrition, inadequate and unsanitary housing and other sociological problems have been shown to have a greater correlation with infant mortality than the number of physicians, or hospitals, or how those physicians and/or hospitals are paid.

The attention given the infant mortality criticisms is even more amazing when one considers that infant mortality accounts for only 2.2 percent of all the deaths in the United States. If the United States had the best infant mortality prevention record in the world, if such things were determinable, that alone would not prove that American health care was the best; similarly, if the United States had the worst infant mortality rate in the world, that would not prove that American health care, as a whole, was poor.

For example, the same United Nations report that contains the much-quoted infant mortality *figures* (not comparisons) also includes mortality rates from four other killers—tuberculosis, pneumonia, bronchitis, and stomach ulcers. Since there are no questions of viability or definition involved, these figures might be more accurately comparable. The table lists mortality figures from 11 countries—Denmark, Finland, France, West Germany, the Netherlands, Switzerland, Japan, Australia, England (including Wales), Sweden and the United States.

In 1967 (the year cited in the 1970 UN report), the United States recorded 3.5 deaths from tuberculosis for every 100,000 citizens. This rate was lower (better) than that reported by seven of the other 10 countries. In fact, Switzerland's rate was twice as high; West Germany's rate was three times as high (as was Finland's); the TB death rate in France was nearly four times as high; the rate in Japan was more than five times as high.

In 1967, the reported death rate from pneumonia in the United States was 28 per 100,000. This rate was only slightly higher than the rates in Denmark and Japan, and lower than the rates in Finland, Australia, Sweden and England. In fact, Sweden (the nation with the "lowest" infant mortality rate) has nearly twice as many deaths from pneumonia as does the United States, and the pneumonia death rate in England is nearly two and one-half times as high as the U.S. rate (66.4, compared to 28.0).

Every one of the other 10 nations in the report has a higher bronchitis death rate than the U.S. In fact, while the U.S. has only 3.2 bronchitis deaths per 100,000 population, the rate in Sweden is twice as high; the rate in Denmark is more than five times as high and the rate in England is nearly 19 times as high!

The United States recorded five stomach ulcer deaths per 100,000 population in 1967. The rate in the Netherlands was just slightly lower (4.5); the rate in six of the 10 nations was worse—including, again, Sweden, Denmark, West Germany, Switzerland and England.

It appears then, that the countries with which the U.S. is so frequently compared unfavorably, on the basis of infant mortality "comparisons," do not fare so well in other comparisons *in the same report.*

It has been suggested that if the infant mortality "comparison" is adequate to prove that American health care is inferior to the care available in the other 10 countries, the reported figures are probably also adequate to prove:

(a) that Sweden has the *best* health system because it has the lowest infant mortality rate;

(b) that Sweden and England have the *worst* health care systems, because each nation had higher death rates than the U.S. in four of five categories cited—more than any of the other nations on the list;

(c) that the Netherlands has the best health system because it has the lowest death rate due to both tuberculosis and pneumonia;

(d) that the United States has the best health system because it has the lowest death rate due to bronchitis;

(e) that France has the best health system because it has the lowest death rate due to ulcer of the stomach;

(f) that Finland and Switzerland have *better* health care systems than the United States, because both have lower infant mortality rates;

(g) that Finland and Switzerland have *worse* health care systems than the United States, because both have higher death rates in three of the four other categories.

Of the nations that hold such mystical allure for the planners, Sweden and England have higher death rates than the U.S. in all four categories above; Finland, Switzerland and West Germany have higher death rates in three of the four categories; Denmark and France have higher death rates in two of the four categories.

Three conclusions may be drawn from the foregoing discussion:

1.   There is not a health care crisis in the United States from the standpoint of deterioration. To the contrary, medical care in the United States improves substantially every year.

2.   Despite the repeated claims of those who would destroy the current American medical system and replace it with some form of socialized medicine, there is not a health care crisis in the United States from the standpoint of comparison with other nations. On the contrary, the United States fares very well in such comparisons.

3.   The attack on the quality of American medical care has been *purposely deceitful.* Those are strong words—stronger than I have used in any other part of this book, though I am obviously convinced that the argument against government medicine is overwhelming from other standpoints as well; therefore, I will cite three considerations that lead me to conclude that the evidence of purposeful deceit is sufficient to warrant such a charge.

A. *Why, if deceit was not intended, did the advocates of national health insurance base their claims of inadequacy of care on a problem that accounts for only two percent of all the deaths in the United States?*

I submit that the primary consideration in that determination was *propaganda value.* Infant deaths arouse emotional response. Reports of bronchitis death statistics simply would not have the same effect. I submit that another reason for the decision to use the infant mortality statistics so extensively was the fact that the reported figure of the U.S. was lower than that of nine other countries in the UN table; a statement that the United States ranks tenth or worse in some category of health care is bound to produce more emotional response than a more accurate comparison based on multiple factors.

B. *Why, if deceit was not intended, did the advocates of national health insurance base their charges on a comparison of figures that were clearly not comparable?*

C. *Finally, if deceit was not intended, why have the advocates of national health insurance*

(1) *failed to disclose to the public the fact that the figures cited are not comparable;* that is, why have the many speakers and writers who have repeated this charge done so without informing their audiences of the factors that make the comparisons unreliable and invalid?

(2) *failed to disclose to the public the disclaimers of comparability that have been published by the sources*—the United Nations and the U.S. Public Health Service?

(3) *failed to disclose to the public that the figures on infant mortality were part of a chart that reported mortality rates from several causes, and that "comparisons" drawn from the other charts would lead to an opposite conclusion?*

It is my opinion that the evidence on the infant mortality question supports—at least inferentially—a conclusion that the advocates of national health insurance have purposely attempted to mislead the American public in an attempt to further their own political goals.

In 1969, *Time* magazine, in a cover story attacking the quality of American medical care (using, as one basis, the infant mortality statistics), stated: "Each year, 27 million Americans go into a general hospital, where they spend an average of 8.2 days . . ."

That intended *criticism,* however, reveals another indicator of the high quality of American medical care. Assuming a population of 200 million (slightly less than actual figures), then only about 13 of every 100 Americans go into a general hospital, for any reason, in a year. This figure includes both maternity cases and persons hospitalized due to accidental injury—neither of which can be attributed to deficiencies in medical care.

In 1968, there were 3,449,000 hospital births. Approximately 20 of every 1,000 women who gave birth had more than one child. Subtracting 69,000 (the number of women having two children), we find that approximately 3,380,000 of the 27 million hospital patients were women having babies. Thus, only 12 of every 100 Americans (24 million) entered a hospital in 1968 for purposes other than having a baby.

Approximately 45 million Americans are accidentally injured each year (*Statistical Abstract of the U.S., 1971*, table 117, page 82). Although many who are not seriously injured are no doubt hospitalized, and many who subsequently die of their injuries are also hospitalized, I will estimate, for the purposes of demonstration, a low figure of only 10.8 million persons hospitalized as the result of accidental injury (this is the number who survived but received either permanent or temporary disability as a result of accidents in 1968: *1971 World Almanac*, Page 68).

This reduces the number of persons hospitalized for illness to approximately 13.2 million—or approximately seven out of every 100 Americans.

Thus, what *Time* is actually saying is that only seven out of every 100 Americans are so ill as to require hospitalization during the course of a year, and that, on the average, they are out again in approximately one week.

Though the assertion is non-scientific, admittedly, I will nonetheless assert that this is a record of which American medicine can be somewhat proud. And be that the case or not, it seems certain that, insofar as serious illness is concerned, there is no medical crisis.

In summary, despite the cries of critics to the contrary, the American citizen continues to enjoy good medical care. He is growing larger and living longer. Many of the diseases that threatened him in the past are being reduced to impotence. He is generally free from illness and able to go about his work. (The average American male visits a physician only 3.8 times a year, and loses only 5.2 days of work each year.)

Of course, there are imperfections in medical care, as there are in other things. There is always room for improvement. But the continued existence of imperfection does not constitute a "crisis," and speakers and writers who use the word should be challenged promptly.

Medical care in the United States today is far better than it has ever been before. Further improvement is desirable, as it always has been and always will be. But *there is no medical crisis.*

5. The Cost "Crisis"

Advocates of national health insurance contend that health care is not only inadequate, but unreasonably expensive. They cry that the cost of care has increased so drastically that most Americans can no longer afford the expense of staying well, and that this high cost creates a medical "crisis" in terms of that care being financially unavailable to the public. The only way to solve that cost "crisis," and thus make the nation's health-care potential truly meaningful, they say, is to assign the job of paying for that care to the government, through a system of national health insurance.

To determine the validity of these contentions, we must consider five questions:

    1.   Has there been a significant increase in the cost of medical and/or health care?

    2.   If there has been a significant increase, has that increase been in line, or out of line, with the general economic pattern in the United States during the period of that increase?

    3.   If there has been a significant increase in health-care costs, is that increase due to the free enterprise system or to other, broader, factors that are not within the control of the current medical/health-care system?

    4.   If there has been a significant increase, has that increase created a situation in which health care costs have made that care

unavailable, or inordinately expensive, to a large segment of Americans?

5. Finally, is it reasonable to conclude that the average American will pay less for his health care under a system of national health insurance? Is it reasonable to conclude that he will pay *more* under such a system?

Clearly, if the United States is to discard a familiar medical system, one which provides good health care (see Chapter 4) in an atmosphere of individual freedom and guaranteed confidentiality, there must be compelling reasons to do so. If the system is to be discarded because of its cost, it must be shown that the cost is unreasonable, that it inhibits access to care, and that another system would be less expensive.

Those who would substitute socialized medicine, or some lesser degree of governmental financing and regulation of medicine, seldom carry the consideration beyond the first question. Has there been a significant increase in the cost of medical care? They answer, using broad general figures, that there has been. Ergo, a cost "crisis." Such a study is insufficient and conclusions from it are misleading.

For example, in asking whether there has been a significant increase in the costs of medical and/or health care, one must consider *two* factors: first, has the *total national expenditure* for health care increased, either in dollar sums or percentages of the gross national product (an interesting exercise for accumulators of statistical minutiae), and secondly, of more valid significance, has there been a substantial increase in the actual number of dollars spent by the average American *individual* to maintain or regain his health?

There is apt to be a considerable difference in the findings, depending on which of the two factors is considered and which is left out of the calculations. The advocate of government medical programs points to an increase in total health care expenditures from $26.4 billion in 1960 to $67.5 billion in 1970, and to an increase in per capita health care expenditures from $183.12 in fiscal 1966 to $256.04 in fiscal 1969—an increase of nearly $75 per person. The truth is, while there was an increase, it was only slightly more than $21 *so far as the average American was concerned* (the per capita *private* health care expenditure rose from $143.44 to $164.81 during the period 1966–69).

A good part of the increased cost is that of the Federal programs promoted by the critics themselves. For example, in the first three full years of Medicare (July, 1966, through June, 1969) the government disbursed $11.2 billion for the hospital insurance portion of the program, and approximately $4.9 billion for the supplementary medical portion. Those who advocated Medicare for the *purpose* of increasing expenditures on health care now complain that health-care expenditures have increased, which is like a man instructing his wife to buy more apples, and then complaining that apples are taking an increased percentage of his income.

Although advocates of national health insurance argue that the Medicare expenses merely replaced funds being spent by the aged themselves ("if they were getting medical care at all"), the facts do not justify such a conclusion. Robert Myers has reported that disbursements for the hospital insurance portion ran 41.1 percent above estimates—due to the increased costs "which, however, were consistent with the general upward trend in prices" and due to "the higher utilization of services than had been assumed."

A good part of the cost was in administrative expense for maintaining the Medicare bureaucracy. During the period 1966–70, for example, administrative expenses for the hospital insurance portion of the program totaled $485 million.

The figure also includes all government spending for pollution control (1971 budget request: $106 million); construction ($89.3 million); non-productive "planning" (the 1971 budget request for Comprehensive Health Planning, which presumably "saves" money by approving or disapproving hospital expansions and equipment purchases, among other things, was nearly a quarter of a billion dollars); Medicaid (1971 request: $2.86 billion); government research programs ($1.03 billion); etc.

It is not the purpose of this report to discuss the merits or demerits of these programs. It *is* my purpose, however, to point out that talk of multi-billion-dollar increases in *total* health expenditures is self-serving and meaningless in terms of discussing whether the individual American is able to meet the cost of staying well.

According to figures compiled by the American Medical Association's Center for Health Services Research and Development, the per capita *private* health expenditure of the average American under age 65 increased approximately $33 between 1966 and 1969

—from $128.04 to $161.84, while the private expenditure for persons aged 65 and older fell approximately $100—from $293.49 to $193.04. Presumably, the $100 burden was removed from the elderly and shouldered instead by the Federal Government, through Medicare. Instead of government spending for the elderly increasing by a corresponding rate of $100, however, Federal spending for this segment of the population soared by $370 per person—from $129.51 to $499.08.

It has been argued by those few liberals who still defend Medicare, despite its 41 percent cost overrun, that the increase was necessary—that obviously this increase must indicate that vast numbers of elderly Americans were in desperate need of medical care before 1965, when the Medicare law was passed, and that the high cost of the program merely proves how many people were doing without care prior to the program. That, of course, is a debatable point. Although there has been clear-cut evidence of increased utilization of medical facilities since Medicare was introduced, the increase is not universal. For example, in the year July 1963–June 1964, prior to Medicare, the average American between ages 65 and 74 visited the physician 6.3 times a year. Similarly, in the earlier period, before Medicare, persons aged 75 and over visited a physician 7.3 times a year; after Medicare was passed the number for both age groups was down to 6.0 times a year (July 1966-June 1967).

It is true, however, that Medicare has resulted in increased demand for care, whether due to prior unmet needs or not. The most striking example is in the great jump in nursing-home admissions. According to the Department of Health, Education and Welfare, the number of nursing-home facilities in the United States increased from 13,514 in 1963 to more than 19,000 in 1967, with an increase in resident patients from 491,397 to 756,239.

Since almost all Americans are covered by private health insurance, it seems unlikely that many persons who actually need medical care go without it. This conclusion is somewhat borne out by government figures, reported later in this chapter, that reveal that the average low-income family in the U.S. spends only $26 less per year on health care than does the upper-income family, which presumably can meet its medical needs. Such evidence indicates that most Americans can and do purchase the health care they actually need, though they may forgo preventive checkups or physician visits for minor ailments. While it may be desirable for all persons to have access to medical comfort for all minor wants as well as major needs, it seems unlikely that the American taxpayer would willingly accept the excessive taxation and reduced quality of care inherent in national health insurance merely to provide non-essential medical services to those few who cannot now afford them.

However, regardless of whether one concludes that the increased Federal spending for Medicare was necessary to provide service to those who needed it, it seems clear that much of the increase in health-care spending was due to the expense of operating government programs, and that the increase in *total* per capita expenditures, while it may or may not be indicative of the cost of meeting need, is certainly not indicative of the extent of increase in the cost of individual purchases of health care.

There are, of course, other factors involved in the increase in total health-care expenditures—increased population, new and more sophisticated medical technology, etc.—but disregarding temporarily the *causes* of increased costs, it seems clear enough, as an observable fact, that *something* has caused an increase in the amount of money spent on health care out of the cumulative American pocketbook.

U.S. News & World Report, for example, on August 10, 1970, reported that *total outlays for medical care in the U.S.* increased from $12.1 billion in 1950 to $67.6 billion (approximately) in 1970. The increase caused the health-care share of the gross national product to increase from approximately 4.5 percent in 1950 to 7.0 percent in 1969.

The Consumer Price Index shows similar increases. Between 1969 and 1970, medical-care costs increased by 7.3 percent. Physician fees increased 8.1 percent; hospital daily charges increased 13.5 percent; dentists' fees rose 5.5 percent; drug prices rose 2.5 percent.

From the foregoing discussion, it can be concluded that (a) *total* national health expenditures—including all the many programs for which the government spends health-care dollars (construction, planning, administration, etc.)—have increased substantially during recent years; (b) costs of individual medical-care components have increased—some substantially (hospital charges), some more moderately; (c) the average number of dollars spent to stay well by the average American under age 65 has increased also, but in far more moderate proportion.

Given that medical costs have increased, it becomes essential to consider whether that increase has been inconsistent with the general economic trend. For example, while it is true that physician fees increased by 8.1 percent during 1970, that figure is valid only when considered in conjunction with the overall increase of 5.5 percent in the consumer price index for all goods and services. The physician, having the same non-medical expenses as his neighbor, had to increase his fees by almost 5.5 percent merely to stay even with inflation and retain the same purchasing power he was earning the year before. The proper figure to be considered in weighing medical cost increases is *the increase of 2.6 percent above the increase in costs of all goods and services,* not the total 8.1 percent increase.

The truth is, the increase in physician fees has been well in line with the general increase in costs and wages during recent years. Robert Myers, in his book *Medicare,* reported that the average annual increase in physician fees during the years 1956 through 1965 (prior to the adoption of the Medicare law) was 3.0 percent, but that the average annual increase in non-medical wages was 3.6 percent.

Government officials anticipated physician-fee increases following the passage of Medicare, which imposed additional paperwork requirements on doctors, necessitating the addition of extra office help and purchase of additional office equipment. Indeed, during the first three years after the law was passed, physician fees increased 5.9 percent (1966), 7.3 percent (1967) and 5.5 percent (1968), but the combined increase was only one percent more than the increase in the general wage level during that period. It must be remembered also that the average wage earner was not incurring the additional overhead expenses that Medicare reports imposed on the physician.

Including the post-Medicare period, 1966–68, in his figures, Myers reported that the average annual increase in physician fees during the 12-year period 1956–68 was actually 0.5 percent *below* the rise in general wages. During that time physician fees went up 3.7 percent a year, and wages increased 4.2 percent each year. *In other words, physicians fell further behind the general income increase with each succeeding year.*

Since the physician must pay 35–40 percent of his fee income for overhead, and provide his own fringe benefits (including insurance, retirement funds, etc.), while wage earners, on the other hand, generally have no overhead and often receive an amount equal to 15–20 percent of their salaries in additional fringe benefits, it is obvious that the physician's "wages" have lagged far behind the wage increases enjoyed by his patients. (The Associated Press, in early 1970, reported that an Indiana physician had to raise his office charges when cost accounting studies revealed that he was netting only 83 cents per patient.)

There are other indices, too:

Department of Labor statistics released at the beginning of 1970 revealed that in the preceding two years the cost of all medical care had increased 12.9 percent, less than such other items as meats, poultry and fish (up 13.6 percent), home ownership (up 18.2 percent), transportation (up 13 percent) and insurance (up 21.4 percent). The increase in medical costs was about the same as the increase in clothing, shoes and restaurant meals.

A report in *Changing Times* magazine, April, 1971, pointed out that the average commodity and service price increase between December, 1967, and December 1970, was 17.2 percent, and that the average increase for the past decade had been 33.3 percent. Although physician fees had risen during that time, the survey revealed that the 10-year increase was approximately the same as, or less than, the increased cost of such items as lettuce, apples, cabbage and tomatoes; domestic help; painting a room; shingling a roof; property insurance; transit fares; auto insurance; movie admissions; college tuition; newspapers; haircuts and women's shampoos. The cost of a tonsillectomy had risen less than the cost of cheese, colas, men's suits and women's dresses.

In other words, the rise, though noticeable and painful to the purchaser, has been a part of the general increase in all prices and wages due to Federal inflationary policies, and has been consistent with the increase in other costs—the purchaser's own income. For example, the *Wall Street Journal*, on January 6, 1970, reported that overall personal income in the United States rose almost 20 percent during the two years 1968 and 1969—the same period during which medical costs rose 12.9 percent.

There have been attempts to deceive the public into thinking that medical-care costs are soaring beyond the scope of normal cost increases. For example, *Fortune* magazine, in January, 1970, claimed that, "The cost of physicians' services and the cost of medical care have risen 50 percent since 1959, while the cost of living has gone up only 20 percent." But medical care consists essentially of services, not goods (as included in cost of living statistics). *U.S. News & World Report*, using figures from the Bureau of Labor Statistics, reported on August 25, 1969, that the cost, not only of medical care but of all services, had risen 50 percent during the previous decade; it was the cost of *commodities* that had increased by 20 percent.

Those who attempt to deceive the public into believing that medical costs have risen disproportionately, neglect to point out that the comparatively small increases in the cost of medical care have taken place during a time when members of the U.S. Senate have increased their own salaries from $22,500 a year to $42,500 a year, the cost of operating the U.S. Congress has risen by 156 percent, the three-cent postage stamp has nearly tripled to eight cents, the penny postcard has become a six-cent postcard, and the average expense of attending a four-year private college has increased by more than 80 percent. Medical-care costs *have* increased —but they have increased far less than many other items during a decade of inflation, and have increased less than the incomes of the citizens who must pay for that care.

Although the costs of medical care are not increasing at anything like the "crisis" rate contended by the planners, they are increasing at an observable rate. In 1970, physician fees increased 2.6 percent more than the cost of all goods and services, and hospital room charges continue to increase. While health care remains a bargain, it becomes less so as costs go up. To determine how to halt the increase in medical costs, we must first learn what is *causing* the increase.

Much of the overall cost increase—the cumulative increase in health-care expenditures—is based on factors over which neither the physician nor the hospital administrator has control. For example, Bernard J. Lachner, Assistant Dean of the College of Medicine at Ohio State University, in an article entitled "The Rising Cost of Health Care," reported that 52 percent of the increase in health spending between 1950 and 1967 was the result either of population growth (18 percent) or new techniques and greater utilization of medical services (34 percent).

The *Social Security Bulletin*, in January, 1969, reported similar figures: $5.9 billion (17.9 percent) of the $32.7 billion increase was attributed to population increase, and $11.1 billion (33.9 percent) to other factors exclusive of a rise in the price of health services. Those who criticize the rising cost of medical care on the basis of overall increases in total national health expenditures, without pointing to the large percentage of the increase that is attributable to population growth, are engaged in a massive deception. Obviously, the 200 million Americans of 1970 spent more for *every* consumable item, including medical care, than did the 150 million Americans of 1950.

Although the majority of the increase in health care costs has been due to factors other than price increases, 48 percent of the additional cost *is* due to the fact that physicians and hospitals charge more each year for their services. Before we decide to scrap the American health-care system as "too expensive," however, we must determine the *causes* of that expense and whether costs would continue at the same (or higher) levels under government medical programs. For convenience, we can study the nature of health care cost increases in two separate categories—charges for physician care and charges for hospital care.

A. Physician Charges

Given that the 1970 increase in physician-service charges was 8.1 percent, and the increase for *all* goods and services was 5.5 percent, we have determined that the average physician had to increase his charges by a corresponding 5.5 percent in order to stay even with the marketplace. What caused him to raise his charges an *additional* 2.6 percent?

There are a number of factors, some of which are inherent in the free-market medical system and some of which are not.

1. INCREASED COST OF OFFICE HELP

Ralph M. Thurlow, senior associate editor of *Medical Economics* magazine, in a February, 1970, article entitled "Office Help: What

It Costs Now," reported that salaries of physicians' aides had increased by a full 11 percent between 1965 and 1967. A study released by the New York regional office of the Labor Department reported a five percent pay increase in office-help salaries in the year April, 1968 to April, 1969.

The typical solo physician has an office staff consisting of one combination Secretary/Girl Friday, a receptionist, a billing clerk, and at least one registered nurse. In some cases the cost of hiring a receptionist or separate billing clerk may be shared by two or more doctors in a private clinic or group practice. A report by the Medical Group Management Association revealed that in early 1970 experienced secretaries were earning up to $125 a week in some areas; receptionists were earning $95 a week, billing clerks $103 a week, and RN's over $140 a week. Labor Department figures indicate even higher salaries: $130 a week for secretaries, $115 for receptionists, $162 for registered nurses.

"Office help costs substantially more now than it did just a few years ago," Thurlow concluded.

It is true, of course, that the increased salaries of ancillary medical personnel are attributable to the free-market system in which American medicine operates. As the demand for competent help increases, the persons who provide that help can ask for—and receive—more pay for their services. It is true, also, that a government-controlled system can prevent that overhead increase by placing a ceiling on the incomes of the more than half a million persons who work in physician offices. That change, however, will require far more than a mere restructuring of the nation's health delivery system; it will require a basic change in the American concept of individual freedom and limited government, and will require a large part of the population to give up the right to advance in income and standard of living, while living costs and the wages of other persons continue to rise.

The obvious danger is that those persons who now provide the vital medical backup services in physician offices will simply opt to work elsewhere, leaving essential health-care positions unfilled. The same is true, of course, if physicians themselves voluntarily elect to hold down the wages of their office personnel in an era of rising costs and wages. Their employees will simply look elsewhere.

If physicians are to continue to provide maximum health-care efficiency, they must continue to offer their employees wage levels consistent with the pay scales for similar work in other offices.

2. ADDITIONAL OFFICE HELP AND ADDITIONAL OFFICE MACHINERY.

"Twenty years ago, I had one girl to answer the phone, do the paper work and assist me," a Maryland physician said recently. "Now I have three people. One answers the phone and does the billing, another handles the paperwork, and another helps me."

The story has been repeated countless times in the offices of physicians in every state. The advent of Medicare, and the increase in third-party payments by private insurance companies and the Blue Cross-Blue Shield plans, have resulted in a proliferation of forms, questionnaires, and reimbursement applications. As the burden of record keeping has become increasingly complex, physicians have been forced to add personnel and equipment (primarily duplicating machines and typewriters) to process the paperwork.

The result has been a substantial increase in overhead costs. National health insurance will multiply the physician's paperwork duties many times. The obvious result will be an even higher overhead expense, and higher charges to be paid either by the individual patient or the bill-paying taxpayer.

3. FEES CHARGED FOR FORMER CHARITY PATIENTS.

The *average* price of physician services is not reflective of higher individual charges alone. For example, if some persons are now charged for medical care who once received it free, the result will be an apparent increase in the average physician charge. This is precisely what has happened as a result of the Medicare program.

In an article entitled "Why Medicare Helped Raise Doctors' Fees," in the September, 1968, issue of *Trans-Action* magazine, Theodore R. Marmor, a member of the Institute for Research on Poverty at the University of Wisconsin and a member of the university's political science department, wrote:

". . . it had been a common practice among physicians to reduce or do away with fees for low-income patients. With Medicare, many poor aged people could now afford to pay, and to pay at a higher level. As one physician in a low-income area wrote in *Medical Economics*, now that he was collecting from the poor, his net yearly income had increased 45 percent. And as one doctor told the *Wall Street Journal*, 'Before Medicare I was charging low-income patients only $4 for house calls because I knew they had limited means. But under Medicare I don't dare give them that lower price or the Medicare people will start reimbursing me at $4 for all claims on the grounds that this is my customary fee. So I have to charge them $6 now.' Just the fact that low-income patients would pay, and be charged, higher rates meant that the average prices of physicians' services would increase."

4. "REASONABLE AND CUSTOMARY" FEES.

Medicare contributed to higher physician fees through the profession's predictable reaction to the law's stipulation that physicians would be paid on the basis of their "usual, reasonable and customary fees." Traditionally, physicians have charged their standard fees only to those patients who could afford them, and have performed their services at reduced rates for persons with lower incomes. Most American patients have long been familiar with this practice of a sliding-fee scale. Medicare's provisions prompted an overall fee increase for several reasons:

(a) The law called the doctor's attention to his "customary" or "average" fee. Strange as it seems, many doctors had not paid much attention to their fee scales in the years following World War II; they had simply worked longer hours and used new medical techniques and, as a result, had seen their incomes increase without an increase in individual charges. The law caused many doctors—faced with the prospect of payment on a "customary fee" basis—to study their customary fees and, if they were too low (often still at World War II scales), to raise them.

(b) Since payment was to be made on the basis of "usual" fees in the community, physicians looked around to see what was the usual fee for service among their fellow physicians, and doctors with lower-than-usual fee scales increased their charges to bring them in line with the neighborhood norms.

(c) Doctors feared future government fee freezes (indeed, the fear *has* since become reality) and thus were prompted to move quickly to establish their fees at a level they could live with for the foreseeable future.

(d) Finally, many physicians believed that only by raising their average fee could they receive sufficient payment from their wealthier patients to allow them to offer reduced charges to the elderly and indigent who, even with Medicare, might have to pay high doctor bills.

Again, it was government medicine, not the free-enterprise system, that caused an increase in physician fees. The rigidity of Congressional guidelines and bureaucratic administration *forced* physicians to increase fees to protect their own incomes and to assure their ability to offer reduced rates to the needy. Increased governmental intervention is likely to have similar results.

Advocates of national health insurance argue, of course, that this part of the problem can be met by imposing ceilings on physician charges and physician earnings. There is no doubt that this alternative is possible, and that the results would be as predicted. But there would be another result, too. For the past quarter-century, British doctors have been fleeing their own country for this one. One of the primary reasons for the exodus has been the limited financial opportunity available to physicians in Britain.

It has been stated that the American physician *must* take what he gets, for there will be no place for him to go in pursuit of a non-regulated system of practice. That is not true. Every practicing physician in America graduated at or near the top of his university class, or was near the top of his class when he entered medical school. He then successfully completed four years of one of the most rigorous educational programs in the country. It is not unreasonable to assume that such men, limited to meager incomes in the practice of medicine, will turn to other fields of endeavor. Though many will continue to practice in response to a "higher calling," many others will refuse to work under government regimentation. The result will be a drastic doctor shortage that will imperil the quality of health care here, as it has done in Britain. Indeed, a 1971 survey of 1,586 practicing physicians, conducted by *Medical Economics*, an independent journal, revealed that a full 35 percent would go into early retirement if national health insurance were enacted; 11 percent said they would go into another profession; 10 percent said they would leave clinical work for teaching or research; five percent said they would go on strike, and four percent said they would leave the United States. The totals are somewhat misleading, since some doctors marked several of the options, but it is clear that a minimum of 35 percent of the doctors surveyed would leave the practice of medicine, and that more than 10 percent are willing to change careers rather than practice under a system of national health insurance. In addition, bright college graduates, faced with the prospect of a potentially meager income in the practice of medicine, might elect not to enter a medical career.

5. MALPRACTICE LIABILITY.

There is yet another major factor in the increase in physician charges during recent years—a proliferation of malpractice lawsuits that has driven physicians' liability insurance rates to staggering heights.

Writing in the May 25, 1970, issue of *Medical Economics*, Stanley Ferber and Bart Sheridan, authors of an article entitled "Who'll Stop Runaway Malpractice Insurance Rates?" described the problem:

—An otolaryngologist in Santa Barbara, California, complains that his annual premium for a malpractice insurance policy has risen from $500 in 1967 to nearly $4,000 by mid-1970.

—An obstetrician-gynecologist in Los Angeles, just starting his practice, has to borrow $4,215 from a local bank to pay for his malpractice insurance premiums.

—A general practitioner in San Diego reports that malpractice protection that cost him $490 in 1966 now costs more than $2,200.

Though the problem is at its worst in California, Pennsylvania and other large states, the malpractice liability crisis is affecting physician fees in every part of the nation. The Illinois State Medical Society, in a booklet entitled "The Physician's Liability in Patient Care," warned member doctors that more than 20 percent of all practicing physicians are sued for malpractice at one time or another during their careers; that 7,000 to 10,000 medical malpractice claims are filed in the United States each year; that the number of major ($10,000 or more) malpractice suits in Cook County (Chicago) had more than tripled in four years—from 49 in 1965 to more than 170 in 1969.

Washington columnist Allan C. Brownfeld has written that claims against physicians are rising 8 to 10 percent a year, with annual premiums for malpractice insurance increasing at a rate of nearly 300 percent a year on the average, and more for doctors in high-risk specialties.

In addition, the problem is complicated by a major increase in the size of settlements and court judgements, which sometimes top $1 million.

There is no consensus as to the cause of the suits (the blame has been placed on "fee-chasing lawyers," a national preoccupation with lawsuits, increased complexity of medical technology), but there *is* certainty as to the effect: higher fees passed along to the patients who must ultimately make up part of the cost of the physician's heavy insurance burden.

"Some doctors," writes Brownfeld, "say they have raised their fees as much as 20 percent during the past year to cover their higher insurance costs."

There is another way in which the abundance of medical malpractice suits has created higher service charges. As physicians concentrate on the avoidance of lawsuits, they become increasingly cautious in their treatment of patients, and the patients usually end up paying unnecessarily for the extra caution. Dr. Carl A. Hoffman, chairman of the American Medical Association's professional liability committee, explained that, "Many doctors will order procedures that actually they feel aren't necessary—tests they wouldn't order on their own family—but they're afraid of omitting a test or a detail which might be held against them in case of a later suit."

"A couple of years ago I'd take off cysts in my office," said a Los Angeles doctor. "Now if I have to do any surgery, I send patients to the hospital. Of course, this adds to the cost of medical care."

A Long Island surgeon said that if he were to discover an abdominal tumor while performing an appendectomy, he would sew up the patient, bring him out of anesthesia, obtain signed consent to perform the additional surgery, and only then operate to remove the tumor. The result is both increased risk for the patient (two operations) and greatly increased cost. But failure to obtain "informed consent" of the patient is a frequent issue in medical malpractice actions.

Another problem stems from increased reliance on second opinions to reinforce medical diagnoses. Dr. William Quinn, a prominent Los Angeles physician, says, "A doctor's greatest comfort during a suit is knowing that a colleague was consulted. Just the other day I saw a patient who needed breast surgery. Since she also had a heart condition I had to call in a heart specialist to confirm that she'd be a reasonable risk for surgery. It's important to have his statement on the record, but it cost the patient an extra consultation fee."

Senator Abraham Ribicoff (D-Connecticut), in his introduction to a study entitled "Medical Malpractice: The Patient vs. the Physician," warned that the proliferation of malpractice lawsuits "threatens to become a national crisis." Ribicoff's assessment is based largely on the effect malpractice suits have had on medical charges. "As the government continues to provide payment for care to millions of Americans," he said, "it is absorbing their share of the increasing cost of malpractice insurance premiums."

We live today in a crisis-oriented society, in which problems are automatically termed "crises," and meet with bursts of frantic activity that are frequently resolved in a series of cries for government funds and government regulation. Yet whether the sudden increase in malpractice lawsuits is merely a solvable problem or truly on the verge of creating a "national crisis," as Ribicoff claims, the effect has been to nudge medical costs upward.

Increased payrolls, larger staffs, expensive new office equipment, Medicare-induced fees for former charity patients, Medicare reimbursement policies, malpractice lawsuits, plus higher rent and increased postage costs—have all had an effect in causing physician charges to rise 2.6 percent faster than the 5.5 percent overall increase in the cost of goods and services. With these factors considered, it seems almost remarkable that physician charges have not increased far more rapidly.

Critics of the free-market medical system contend that increased medical costs stem from the system itself, with physicians greedily increasing their fees to take advantage of increased demands for care. The facts indicate that physicians have been remarkably restrained in increasing fees to reflect the additional costs that they must bear in order to provide their services.

Of the factors that have caused the rise in physician charges, one —increased payrolls—could be alleviated by passage of a national health insurance law, and then only if the law provided for the virtual enslavement of ancillary medical personnel by ordering the half-million clerks and nurses in doctor's offices to work for limited wages.

National health insurance would likely *increase* the problems in the other areas. The extensive nationwide bureaucracy that would be established to direct such a program would create stacks of new paperwork to be taken care of by physicians and their office aides (GPs in Britain must fill out and submit more than 20 separate forms, ranging from immunization reports to applications for space in hospital maternity wards). To continue to provide the same amount of service, physicians would have to increase their staffs even more—and each new employee would require supporting office equipment.

With everybody in the nation covered by a blanket of government health insurance, charity care would disappear and the nation's taxpayers would have to reimburse doctors for care that they now give either free or at greatly reduced rates.

There *are* solutions to these problems, but these solutions obviously do not lie in the direction of further government intervention. In at least three areas—staff and equipment requirements, fees for former charity patients, and cost increases resulting from Medicare reimbursement policies—it seems that the best way to hold costs down would be to *reduce* the degree to which government already intervenes in the practice of medicine.

In 1970, *Medical Economics* magazine printed the results of a nationwide survey of 3,000 families to determine the public's reaction to medical charges. The magazine reported that 76 percent thought the family doctor *deserves* what he earns, and another 15 percent thought he deserved *even more.* Asked if they thought the doctor's fees were too high, 73 percent answered that the charges were about right, and another five percent thought they were too low.

Clearly, the "uproar" over physician fees is not coming from the patients—or at least not from the big majority of patients. Instead, the complaints are coming from a handful of patients and from vocal liberals in the press and in politics who are trying to convince Americans that they ought to get upset about physician fees "because everybody else is upset." The goal, of course, is national health insurance, a goal pursued more for reasons of social philoso-phy than for any real concern over a "crisis" in American medicine.

B. Hospital Charges

The most noticeable—and most disturbing—element of the in-crease in medical costs has been the rapid rise of daily charges for hospitalization. In 1970, the cost of hospital-room charges in-creased by 13.5 percent—more than 50 percent faster than the charge for physician services. Since hospitals account for more than 37 percent of health care expenditures (compared to 19.6 percent for doctors' services), the increase has been of major national con-cern.

Critics of the private medical system contend that costs will be reduced by the enactment of national health programs; the facts indicate that just the opposite would be true. Although the United States has approximately 12 times as many private, non-government hospitals (5,000) as Federal Government hospitals (415), and ap-proximately eight times as many private beds (1,300,000 versus 170,000), the amount of money spent for care in private hospitals is only *six* times as great (23.2 percent of total health-care expendi-tures, compared with 3.9 percent spent in government hospitals).

The conclusion that hospitalization costs *more* under government medicine is borne out by studies in New Orleans and Detroit that revealed longer average hospitalization stays (and thus higher costs per illness) in government hospitals (See Chapter 14). Nonethe-less, hospital costs *have* risen and it is essential to determine if the cost increases are the fault of the free enterprise system or are due to other factors.

The operation and maintenance of a modern hospital facility is a highly complex procedure. For example, while hospitals have frequently been referred to as "hotels for the sick," there is quite an amazing difference between hospitals and hotels—and a corre-sponding difference in costs. While the average hotel has six times as many guests as employees, the average hospital has 2.5 times as many employees as patients. According to Blue Cross statistics, a hospital requires 14 times as many employees as a hotel of compara-ble size.

While hotels provide the use of a room, housekeeping services, utility and maintenance services, linens and laundry facilities, hospitals provide each of these services *plus* delivery of all meals to the patient's room, preparation of special diets, 24-hour-a-day nursing care, drugs and medications, surgery facilities, physical therapy facilities and expensive lifesaving equipment.

With such a widespread range of services, hospitals are subject to many factors that tend to increase the cost of operation. Among the more important:

1. INFLATION.

Like other consumers, hospitals are affected by the inflationary economic trends that have beset the United States in recent years. In fact, inflation strikes the average hospital *more* severely than many other businesses, due to the large number of items that must be stocked to provide satisfactory service.

Hospitals are large-scale consumers of many goods, ranging from bed linens to the beds themselves, and to television sets, telephone equipment, food, serving trays, silverware, and complicated medical equipment. As a result, inflation—a direct outgrowth of government economic decisions—has had a significant effect on hospital charges. H. E. "Sandy" Hamilton, director of New Orleans' famed Ochsner Foundation Hospital, has pointed out that it now costs approximately $500 to replace a hospital bed purchased 10 years ago for $150. According to a Blue Cross study, the cost of linens has increased by approximately six percent; the cost of medical, pharmaceutical and surgical supplies has risen by approximately 12 percent.

In all, it is estimated that the average hospital purchases more than 10,000 items—and the continually higher cost it must pay for each purchase is reflected in increased charges for patient care.

2. PAYROLL.

Ironically, though it is organized labor that provides the most vocal criticism of hospital charges, much of the recent increase is directly attributable to the dramatic hike in hospital wages during recent years.

At Pennsylvania Hospital, in Philadelphia, for example, wages for service workers such as maids and cooks, went up by 43 percent between 1969 and 1971. Salaries for X-ray technicians increased by 39 percent, as did the pay for licensed practical nurses. Wages for registered nurses went up 25 percent; the pay rate for clerical help increased by 42 percent. The effect of such increases on hospital-room charges is obvious when one considers that salaries and wages account for 70 percent of a hospital's overhead, compared with approximately 28 percent in industry (hospitals sell services, not goods, and salaries make up the chief expense of providing personal service).

While industry can absorb wage and salary increases and make up the higher overhead through increased production, hospitals have little opportunity either to increase production or reduce salaries through mechanization and automation, since patients demand highly personalized care in American hospitals. In fact, there is frequent insistence that hospitals *increase* the amount of personal service they provide, and decrease the use of impersonal time-saving and cost-cutting procedures.

Hospital salaries are frequently higher than those in industries of comparable size, as a result of the demand for *skilled* workers in many hospital functions, such as nursing and technology. Approximately one-third of all hospital employees are classified as skilled workers, compared to only one out of six, for example, in the auto manufacturing industry. Technological developments in recent years have required nurses to come to their jobs equipped with greater skills than ever before. This new demand has required more specialized (and more costly) training, and has enabled nurses to demand higher wages for their work. Traditionally underpaid, nurses have seen their salaries tripled in the past 25 years.

Dr. George Graham, former President of the American Hospital Association, has estimated that administrative and general man-hours in hospitals increased 15 percent during the first year of Medicare. Now, other factors may combine to push hospital wages —and hospital charges—still higher. Hospital employees are now covered by Federal minimum wage laws for the first time. Since wages form the bulk of hospital overhead, pay increases resulting from this new extension of Federal regulation will be reflected in higher daily room charges passed on to patients.

Labor leaders in Pennsylvania have managed to push through

their state legislature a new law permitting state employees (including hospital workers) to go on strike. John F. Worman, Executive
Vice President of the Pennsylvania Hospital Association, has predicted that the law could result in hospital charges increasing by as
much as another $30 per day. There is a good possibility that
similar laws will be enacted in other states as well.

3. OVERUTILIZATION.

Third-party payment—payment either by Federal or private insurance plans—has been a major cause of the increase in hospital-
care expenditures. When somebody else pays the bill, the patient
simply has no financial motivation to speed up the healing process
—a conclusion borne out by the excessive number of days spent in
the hospital by patients in VA and Public Health Service facilities
(see Chapter 14) and in hospitals in other countries in which the
government picks up the tab (see Chapter 10).

Dr. George E. Shambaugh, Jr., a professor at Northwestern
University, described the problem in a privately published booklet
entitled "The Cost of Medical Care and What You and I Can Do
About It":

"Medicare and Medicaid . . . are costing three or four times as
much as the government planners expected," he wrote. "One reason is that the patient, with all his bills paid for him, lacks any
incentive to leave the hospital as soon as he is able to. We saw this
in the VA hospitals where a fenestration operation required an
average of eight weeks of hospitalization, compared to eight days
in a private hospital. Another reason is that patients want to be
hospitalized for X-rays and other diagnostic tests which their insurance will not pay for on an outpatient basis."

Private health insurance plans, which often pay only if a patient
is hospitalized, have also created expensive overuse of hospitals. In
mid-1970, Dr. Edward R. Pinckney, a Berkeley, California, specialist, told a Senate subcommittee, "If a patient, because of the benefits
of his health plan, is entitled to receive medical care in a hospital
with no out-of-pocket expense to himself, he will rarely, if ever,
prefer to pay some of his own money for the identical service in his
doctor's office.

"The health plan, by paying fully for medical care within a hospital, and only partially, if at all, for outside care, really leaves no option open to the patient or his physician. Both are logically forced to select the place for diagnosis and treatment where the patient will not be directly responsible for the cost of his care."

A number of prominent physicians have urged the private insurance industry to make policy changes to permit office treatment and thus reduce medical-care costs. "I contend that sickness and accident insurance in the form that most of it is written now constitutes the most significant driving force in the escalation of medical costs," charged Dr. Lester Karotkin of Houston, a former president of his county medical society. Dr. Karotkin has urged insurance companies to offer the public simple disability policies, with fixed payments, regardless of whether a patient is treated in a hospital, at home, or in a physician's office, and regardless of whether he recuperates in a hospital or at home in his own bed.

4. GOVERNMENT.

To some extent, hospital costs have gone up as a result of what government medicine already exists.

In 1969, the administrator of a large Texas hospital informed officials of the Social Security Administration that his hospital was being forced to stop providing services under the Medicare program, because the program was threatening to ruin the hospital financially. The problem arose over a Medicare policy of compensating participating hospitals only for actual care costs. The Texas hospital, like others, charged on a basis of actual cost plus a prorated share of the overhead for providing such essential services as maternity and nursing facilities, costly equipment, etc. Because of the lower payment for Medicare patients, the hospital was faced with the apparent necessity of increasing the overhead cost borne by other, non-Medicare patients.

Located in the Lower Rio Grande Valley, with a large number of moderate-income patients, the hospital decided it could not increase the costs to its other patients (and could not absorb the loss), so it simply pulled out of the program. Other hospitals have undoubtedly elected to pass the buck, literally, in the form of higher day charges for non-Medicare patients (meaning, of course, for the great majority of Americans).

In addition, hospitals, too, have been hard hit by the plethora of Federal regulations surrounding Medicare and Medicaid. Paperwork has multiplied rapidly, and hospitals have been forced to increase clerical and administrative staffs to meet the added burden.

5. TECHNOLOGICAL ADVANCEMENT.

Much of the increased spending on health care is attributable to the availability of new medical techniques—advancements that frequently mean life for persons who would have died without the sophisticated new equipment in medical offices and hospitals.

Philip Wagner wrote of a case that illustrates this point in the *Philadelphia Bulletin,* of July 8, 1970: "A man of 65 suffered a heart block last winter . . . ," he wrote. "Fifteen years ago, he would have been condemned to spend the rest of his life an invalid with his pump barely clunking along. Today, a device called a pacemaker is installed under his chest muscle, connected with the interior of his heart by means of electrodes threaded through his jugular vein and supplies the heart-beats his own heart misses." (Ironically, Wagner used the case to complain of the high cost of the care.)

Dr. George C. Roche III, President of Hillsdale College and formerly on the staff of the Foundation for Economic Education, discussed the same point in an article in *Private Practice* magazine:

". . . over one-third of the total medical expenditures during the past 20 years have been due to an increase in the quantity and/or quality of services rendered to the typical patient—indicating better service, rather than higher prices," Dr. Roche wrote.

"One study, measuring health care expense and service between 1950 and 1967, concludes, 'After allowing for population growth, people in 1967 were enjoying $11.1 billion each year of services beyond what they had been receiving in 1950.' The techniques that have come into common use during the past 20 years of rapid medical advance are often costly. The tests common to the practice of medicine today are far more numerous and complex than 20 years ago. The equipment in use is often far more sophisticated.

"I would suspect," Dr. Roche says, "that there are few objections to the higher costs of health care from the ranks of those who are alive today because of the techniques and equipment which have come into existence since 1950."

Dr. Shambaugh describes the effect of technological advance:

"One reason [for the increase in medical care costs]," he writes, "is the rapid advance of scientific medicine with the addition of new, valuable, but expensive diagnostic tests. An example is the new method of X-raying the inner ear and hearing nerve called polytomography. This requires an apparatus . . . costing $75,000, plus $25,000 to install. . . . With it we are now able to diagnose tumors of the hearing nerve as small as a pea, whereas before we could not make the diagnosis until such a tumor had become as large as a small lemon and had reached the brain. Today by polytomography we can see defects or fixation of parts of the ossicular chain that carries sound from the eardrum to the hearing nerve, and such defects can be repaired. We are able now, with polytome X-ray studies, to diagnose the early beginnings of otosclerosis *even before the hearing begins to fail,* and we have a method for retarding or arresting the progressive loss of hearing. The problem is that only six examinations a day can be made by the polytome X-ray apparatus, and the least that can be charged for this study to pay for its operation and to amortize the cost of the apparatus and installation is $60. This is quite expensive. But the *benefits* for the patient in diagnosing life-threatening tumors and hearing losses that can be prevented or cured, far outweigh the cost of the examination."

Blue Cross illustrated the financial impact of this lifesaving technology in a fact sheet entitled "The Simple Facts About Hospital Costs." "A hospital, preparing for open heart surgery, invested $75,000 in facilities, equipment and personnel before admitting the first patient for surgery," the report said. The fact sheet pointed out that each heart pump machine costs a hospital $15,000; that each sterilizer costs $17,000; that each cobalt X-ray machine costs more than $80,000; that a linear accelerator costs in excess of a quarter of a million dollars. Even a surgical microscope costs $2,500. "Such equipment saves lives and shortens hospital stays but costs must be allocated among all patients, or be underwritten by grants or gifts."

Because of technological advances, the report said, "More people go to hospitals for treatment; many are now able to walk out . . . *cured of ailments which once were incurable.*"

Although this medical progress has been partly responsible for the increase in daily room charges, it has also reduced treatment and recuperation time, so that although daily costs have increased substantially, the average patient pays only slightly more per illness. For example, the Blue Cross report points out that in 1947 the average duration of hospitalization for pneumonia was 16 days. At a rate of $10 a day, the 1947 patient paid $160 for his hospital care. In 1966, hospital costs were up to $40 a day, but medical progress had reduced the average stay for a pneumonia patient to only five days. Thus the total cost was $200—an increase of only $40, offset by the patient's ability to return to the earning of an income a full 11 days sooner.

In 1947, the average appendicitis patient was hospitalized for two full weeks, for a total cost of $140. By 1966, the average duration of an appendicitis hospitalization had been reduced to four days. The total cost for hospitalization in 1966 was only $20 more than in 1947, and the patient was returned to his employment 10 days sooner.

Dr. Shambaugh also discussed the effects of technological advancement:

"If we go back to the depression years, when the new Wesley Memorial Hospital (in Chicago) opened its doors on Pearl Harbor Day, we find that a two-bed room cost the patient $6 a day . . . In that year (1941) the doctors in this office helped to develop the first successful operation for restoring hearing in progressive deafness, the fenestration operation for otosclerosis. In 1940, the charge by your doctors in this office for a complete initial history and examination, including hearing tests, was $25. The minimum charge for a fenestration operation by the senior doctor was $500, but this operation also cost the patient eight days in the hospital and three or four weeks away from work.

"Today, 28 years later, we charge exactly the same $25 for our complete initial history and examination, including hearing tests. But, we have added two additional tests to this examination, the speech reception and discrimination tests; we have better (and far more expensive) sound-proof testing rooms, while the salaries of our nurses who take the history and audiometrists who do the hearing tests have increased by 200 to 400 percent. All of these increased costs of operation have been absorbed by the doctors at no additional cost to the patient.

"Today, 28 years later, we have a better operation to restore normal or near-normal hearing in patients with otosclerosis: the stapes operation. The minimum charge for this better operation by the same senior doctor, including the first year of post-operative care, is $525. But this improved method requires only three days instead of eight in the hospital and an average of one week instead of three or four away from work, so that actually the total cost to the patient with otosclerosis is *less* today to have his hearing restored through surgery than in 1940."

Critics of increased hospital costs generally overlook the fact that the actual cost to a patient is the per diem charge *times* the number of days in the hospital. To the advocate of national health insurance, the crucial point in Dr. Shambaugh's illustration is the $25, or 5 percent, increase in the cost of the operation. In truth, the crucial points are (a) the improved nature of the operation procedure, and (b) the *actual reduced cost* as a result of the shorter recuperation time.

"What really matters is not the cost per day but the total cost of the illness," writes Alex Gerber, a prominent California surgeon and author. ". . . It is an axiom that the sooner a doctor can send a patient home from the hospital, without undue risk, the better for all concerned. Patients usually thrive better at home; they go back to work earlier and the hospital frees a bed for someone else. Yet the short stay is most costly per day. That is because a patient uses most of the hospital's costly ancillary services at the beginning of his stay. That is when he uses the operating room, X-ray equipment, and labs, and when he requires intensive nursing care. Later on, as he recovers, he uses far fewer of these services. On a long stay, these costs average out over many days; on a short one, they can be averaged only over fewer days and thus raise the cost per day. Thus an efficient short-stay hospital has a higher per diem rate than an inefficient one, but the cost to the patient is generally lower. A seven-day stay at $75 costs $525; a five-day stay at $85 is $100 less!"

Dr. Shambaugh used an illustration based on a fenestration operation to prevent deafness. Millions of Americans are aware of similar advances in open-heart surgery and kidney dialysis procedures that are costly, but which save lives and, in the long run, money.

The increase in hospital charges is undeniable, but it is primarily the result of factors either not attributable to the nature of the present medical system (except insofar as the present system is *not* entirely a free enterprise system—that is, insofar as the system is

susceptible to Medicare administrative policies, governmental economic policies, and Federally-enforced union wage pressures), or
to factors that are, simply, the price one must pay for the medical
advancement (that is, the cost of new medical equipment).

Bernard Lachner made the point well:

"When we talk of costs being too high," he said, "one of the
items usually lacking in such pronouncements is a basis of comparison. If costs are 'too high' they must be compared to the cost of
some other type of service, or to the same service at some previous
time. The hospital service of today is not the hospital service of
yesterday. None of us want it to be. The hospital of today is no
longer supported by charity. The idea that hospitals can be run by
retired physicians, ministers, or someone's nephew, or by anyone
else not possessing management skills, is as foreign to most hospitals today as it is to any multi-billion-dollar institution or industry.

"A comparison of hospitals with hotels or any other segment of
our economy is senseless. Caring for the sick and injured is in no
way similar to manufacturing and retailing commodities. We have
never had any person present themselves at our doors, at any hour,
on any day, and ask for anything less than the very best we had to
offer. No January sales, no discount services, no specials, no sec-
onds—they aren't interested in coming back tomorrow or next
week. The very best we have, at any hour, any day, whether it is
an upset stomach, a toe cut in a lawn mower, an auto accident, a
prison riot, the birth of a baby, elective surgery, diagnostic care, or
a terminal cancer.

"This attitude is shared by all of us when it comes to our own
health."

Those who demand a new health-care system in the United States
frequently base their claims of a cost crisis on assertions that the cost
of health care—regardless of its justification and/or its comparability to income levels and other cost increases—is too high for health
care to be available to the citizen. The facts, however, lead to the
opposite conclusion: health care in the United States remains an
extremely good bargain.

According to figures published in the February 21, 1969, issue
of *Time* magazine, approximately 27 million Americans are hospitalized each year, with an average expense of $530, half of which
is covered by insurance. *In other words, the average American taxpayer*

is hospitalized only once every seven and one-half years, and the out-of-pocket expense for the care he receives and the time spent in the hospital is only about $265, not including his insurance premium payments.

The Social Security Administration's Bureau of Research and Statistics reported in June, 1970, that in the years 1966–69, the average American, age 65 and older, spent only $163 out of his own pocket for medical care; the average citizen under age 65 spent only $98 a year out of his own pocket for medical care—at a time when the median income level in the U.S. was in excess of $8,600.

More recent figures, released at the beginning of 1971 by the U.S. Bureau of Labor Statistics, present similar findings. The Bureau's official estimates for 1969 indicate that total medical-care costs, for a family of four, ranged from an average of $539 for families with low-scale budgets (approximately $5,300 in total annual family consumption) to $543 for moderate-budget families ($8,000 annual consumption), and $565 for high-budget families (approximately $11,000 annual consumption). The figure includes the cost of hospitalization and surgical insurance premiums, a supplementary major medical insurance policy for "high-budget" families, doctors' visits, dental and eye care, drugs, etc.

The nature of the bargain is even more evident when considered as a portion of the family's total yearly expenditures for goods and services. The low-budget family, according to the bureau's report, spends about 10 percent of its consumption (not necessarily its total income, since part of that income will go into savings or investment) on medical and health care; the middle-income or moderate-budget family spends approximately 7 percent of its annual consumption for medical care; for high-income families, medical and health care consumes only five percent of total non-investment spending. Compare this with the national health insurance program in Germany, in which every worker is taxed a full 10 percent of his *total income* for health care.

Overall figures for 1967, reported by the U.S. Department of Commerce and the Health Insurance Institute, produced similar data. Medical-care expenses, including the cost of health insurance premiums, totaled slightly over $33 billion—6.7 percent of total consumer expenditures. By contrast, food and alcohol accounted for 22.3 percent of consumer spending; housing accounted for 14.4 percent; household operation, 14.2 percent; transportation (primarily automobile purchase and maintenance), 12.9 percent; and clothing and jewelry, 10.3 percent. In fact, the average American paid only slightly more to stay well than he paid for recreation —6.2 percent. (It is interesting to note that the average American paid 1.9 percent of his consumer expenditures, or 28 percent of what he spent for medical care, for tobacco, and that he spent twice as much to own and maintain an automobile as he did to maintain his own health.)

The *Social Security Bulletin* for January, 1970, also confirms the current health bargain received by American citizens. The *Bulletin* reports that total per capita private consumer expenditures for all health services and supplies in 1968 totaled $162.65, including that portion paid by insurance. Not only was the figure far below the estimated individual health costs under national health insurance (see Chapter 10), it also revealed a reduction in actual individual health care costs since 1965, when the expenditure figure was $169.78, and 1966, when it was $170.78.

Given the relative importance of maintaining one's health, it seems evident that the costs of medical care are indeed reasonable.

Critics who claim that the average citizen cannot meet the cost of staying well, either (a) ignore the fact that most Americans are covered by private insurance, or (b) claim that private insurance simply doesn't cover enough of the costs of illness. Again, the facts are quite different.

According to 1968 data from the Health Insurance Institute, 89 percent of all Americans under age 65 have private hospital insurance. Even when the aged are included in the figures, 85 percent of the population is covered.

Nor is the coverage only for the costs of hospitalization. In 1968, just under 170 million Americans (including 10 million aged 65 and older) owned private insurance to meet hospital costs. Nearly as many (156 million) were covered for surgical expenses, and approximately 65 percent (130 million) had coverage for regular medical expenses. In addition, approximately 67 million had major medical ("catastrophic") insurance protection, and nearly 63 million had disability income protection.

Insurance picks up the tab for a good portion of the average American's health-care expenses. According to the 1971 *Statistical Abstract of the U.S.* (page 64, table 82), private health insurance paid for 74 percent of all private hospitalization expenses in 1968, and paid nearly 40 percent of the expense of physician services. In all, private health insurance benefit payments in 1968 totaled more than $12 billion, well over double the coverage 10 years earlier.

It is important to remember that insurance is intended solely to *ease* the burden of health-care costs, by making it possible to meet medical expenses without severe financial hardship. Insurance was never meant to pay for all of the cost of all medical care. The cost of such first-dollar coverage would be prohibitive—and for the average American would represent a poor allocation of his assets, since hospitalization occurs so infrequently, and the accumulation of financially crippling health expenses, though not rare, is uncommon.

Private insurance, however, does do a good job of protecting the average citizen against unusually high medical expenses. With the cost of medical care increasing only slightly more than the cost of all goods and services during the past year, and the average middle-income American family devoting only 7 percent of its annual spending for health maintenance, it is clear that American medical care is still a handsome bargain.

If medical costs continue to increase, the inevitable result must be a greater expenditure by the individual who is served by the health-care system. Under a free enterprise system, the added cost is borne only by the patient, as he uses the service; under national health insurance, the increased cost would be reflected in increased taxation for everybody. (Under the American taxation system, with its write-off and deduction provisions that favor upper-bracket taxpayers, the bulk of the added cost will likely be shouldered by persons with low- and middle-level incomes.)

Gunnar Myrdal, the Swedish economist, described the potential results of such a program in an article in *Nation's Business* (April, 1971):

"In Sweden, a person earning $10,000 a year pays up to 46 percent in direct national and local income taxes, plus another 15 to 20 percent in sales taxes and other levies. A Swede making $20,000 a year pays up to 54 percent in income taxes, with numerous other taxes heaped on top of that. A value-added tax on appliances and large items such as cars or boats amounts to 15 percent of the cost of the item.

"As welfare benefits have expanded and taxes have gone steadily higher, the Swedes have been beset by fearful inflation . . .

"After years of constantly cheapening money, Sweden has become a very expensive country to live in, or visit."

Sweden's experience is not unique (see Chapter 10). The evidence in other nations with national health insurance and broad-scale welfare programs indicates that a similar prospect is in store for the United States if this country pursues similar policies.

Rather than expressing unnecessary concern over the cost of medical care, the nation's politicians, who would replace free enterprise medicine with expensive national health insurance programs, should consider that the average American—who would pay heavily in increased taxes to support these government medical plans—is already spending almost seven times as much to pay his taxes as he spends to pay his medical bills. The Tax Foundation, Inc., researching expenditures of workers earning $10,000 a year, found that out of a $40-a-day wage, taxes will consume $13.05, compared with only $1.90 spent on medical care. Of that amount, $8.70 (4.5 times as much as the medical care expense) is taken by the Federal Government. In fact, the Foundation reported, the $10,000-a-year employee works two hours and 37 minutes of every eight-hour workday just to pay his taxes—a figure that will increase considerably if Congress enacts a multi-billion-dollar national health insurance program.

6. The Doctor Shortage

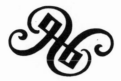

In February, 1970, Assistant HEW Secretary Roger Egeberg declared that the national shortage of physicians, nurses and technicians had reached a state of crisis.

Dr. Egeberg is not alone in the cry for more doctors. As *Medical News Report*, a generally conservative publication, put it: "There's almost universal agreement no problem concerning health care delivery can be solved satisfactorily until the health manpower shortage is alleviated."

To proclaim the existence of a shortage of anything is to presuppose the existence of a figure at which the shortage would cease to exist. The question then becomes: If there is a doctor shortage in the United States, how has the existence of that shortage been determined? In relation to what? The question is more than academic. The general cry of a doctor shortage leaves an implication that must be defended or the charge dropped, for if there *is* a shortage of medical personnel, then obviously the American public is receiving sub-standard medical care (or at least sub-optimal medical care).

First, it might be helpful to consider whether the United States has a shortage of doctors in relation to other countries of the world.

One might suppose that the greater mobility of the American public (our ability to travel farther, and more quickly, in order to

obtain medical care) would indicate a need for fewer doctors per
capita in the United States than in other nations, yet the United
States has *more* doctors per capita than any of the major European
nations to which our health care system is so frequently compared.

The doctor-potential patient ratio in this country is also impressive in comparison with the past. In 1960, there was one physician
for every 712 persons in the United States; a decade later, at the
end of 1969, there was one physician for each 640 persons.

According to Dr. Egeberg, the shortage involves more than
physicians; the "crisis," he says, is one of "medical personnel," a
far broader term encompassing allied health services, such as optometry, osteopathy, nursing and dentistry.

Just how many are not enough?

At the beginning of 1970, there were 328,000 medical doctors
in the United States, of whom 303,000 were in active medical
service. By the end of that year the number of physicians had
increased to 338,000. There are approximately 114,000 dentists in
the United States; more than 135,000 pharmacists; 680,000 registered nurses; 345,000 licensed practical nurses; 800,000 aides,
orderlies and attendants; 14,000 optometrists; 55,000 chiropractors; 204,000 medical and dental technicians—in all, according to
the U.S. Department of Commerce, more than 3.6 million persons
in the health care field.

If one doctor for every 640 persons is not enough; if 3.6 million
health care workers are not enough—how much *is* enough? It
seems self-evident that the answer is simply "enough to do the job."

Yet the figure is not easily determined. For example, the 1967
report of the President's National Advisory Commission on Health
Manpower claimed the existence of a doctor shortage while reporting some revealing statistics:

"From 1955 to 1965, while the population increased 17 percent
and the number of active physicians increased 22 percent, professional nurses in practice increased 44 percent, registered X-ray
technologists increased 56 percent, and clinical laboratory personnel increased 70 percent. In the same period, dentists increased 13
percent, but the number of dental assistants rose by 32 percent and
dental hygienists by 54 percent . . .

"While physicians in private practice increased 12 percent between 1955 and 1965, 'physician-directed' services rose by 81 percent."

Not only did the increase in physicians and paramedical personnel far outpace the increase in population, according to the report: "Present trends indicate that in the coming decade the growth of health services will far outpace the growth of the population." (As predicted, since 1965 the number of physicians has increased three times as fast as the national population.)

What then leads the Commission, from such findings, to the conclusion that "the 'physician shortage' will in all probability continue to worsen"? The answer lends considerable insight into the true nature of the so-called crisis.

"There is inadequate health care for the disadvantaged," the report states. "There are shortages of entry points for the patient into the medical care system, and of personal contact with the physician who usually provides this entry . . . (the shortages are) related to the way in which health personnel are organized . . . we believe that changes in the health care system are . . . essential . . ." In other words, the Commission bases its claim of a doctor shortage not on an actual shortage of doctors, but on the panelists' disagreement with the way those doctors perform their services; on a disagreement with the system—not an unusual sentiment when one considers that the commission, appointed by President Johnson, included several outspoken advocates of government medicine.

The Commission, a major source of the current claims of "doctor shortage," clearly admitted the health care professions' ability to meet patient needs:

"The health sector has demonstrated during the past decade its ability to respond to increased demand. While the supply of physicians and dentists has not responded rapidly to increased demands for health care [author's note: a few pages earlier the report had stated that the number of physicians had increased five percent faster than the population], the supply of nurses and auxiliary personnel has expanded remarkably. Furthermore, the lead time for the training of health personnel—with the exception of physicians, dentists and nurses—is relatively short; thus a rapid response to rising demands is possible.

"Because physicians have rapidly increased their use of auxiliary personnel, diagnostic equipment, laboratory facilities, etc., services provided under the direction of physicians have increased far more rapidly than has the number of physicians. If the 'productivity' trends of the last decade continue, the output of medical services per physician will increase by 50 percent between 1965 and 1975.

"Even under the most pessimistic assumptions, the growth in the supply of physicians is expected to keep pace with population between now and 1975. Given the expected increase in output per physician, there will be at least a 50 percent increase in the per capita supply of physician-directed medical services. Moreover, hospital services, which complement and sometimes substitute for those of the physician, will also increase more rapidly than population."

Clearly the Commission's *findings*—findings that are never publicized—completely refute the existence of a doctor shortage, or a shortage of health care personnel, now or in the foreseeable future.

The report, which is widely cited as the basis of "doctor shortage" claims, actually found and reported just the opposite: while there may be some question as to the optimum utilization of the physician population, there is not, according to the Commission's findings, a shortage of doctors or a shortage of medical personnel.

Harvard Professor Nathan Glazer, in an article entitled "Paradoxes of Health Care," also wondered how many doctors would be enough:

"The case is overwhelming," he said. "Between 1955 and 1965, while population increased 17 percent, medical auxiliary personnel increased 63 percent. That should have made a difference—but, as we have seen, by the later date there was no let-up in projected shortages for the present and the future. If we estimate shortage by some standard established by a professional group as to how much of some kind of personnel is needed, there is indeed a shortage (but) if we estimate shortages on the basis of health in well-served and poorly-served areas, the matter becomes more obscure."

Glazer then quotes William N. Hubbard, to make his point:

"In the United States," Hubbard said, "the ratio of physicians to population varies from 188/100,000 in New York to 93/100,000 in Wisconsin, *with little difference in the general health status of the two states* . . . During World War II there was a massive exodus of physicians from (civilian practice) in 1942, and a sudden return at the end of the war. *These shifts did not affect statistical measures of trends in general health"* (emphasis by Professor Glazer).

In other words, just as there is no doctor shortage in terms of the ability of the number of physicians to keep pace with population growth, neither is it apparent that so-called surpluses or shortages of doctors have a significant effect on the health of the public, so long as each state has a certain minimum number of practitioners. Based on comparisons with New York, Wisconsin obviously has (in Hubbard's example) a doctor shortage. Yet the effect of that shortage certainly does not bear out the existence of a "crisis" in Wisconsin.

The question: "How many doctors are required?" is further clouded by a study by health planner Robert M. Sigmond, also quoted by Glazer.

Sigmond asked dozens of physicians this question: "Suppose this country faced a national emergency like a long world war that required your region to contribute as many physicians, nurses and other health workers as possible. Suppose further that you were placed in charge of the health services in your region . . . Would you be able to contribute any of the region's physicians, surgeons, nurses and other health workers for national emergency service, without impairing the quality of the health service provided in your region?"

Sigmond reported that, "Every single individual whom I questioned believed that if he could achieve complete cooperation and commitment, health manpower in the region could be substantially reduced without impairing quality of care and without adverse effect on the people's health. The unanimity of response was striking.

"Even more striking were these physicians' responses with respect to the amount of reduction in health manpower that could be achieved without reducing the quality or effectiveness of service. When asked to estimate the proportion of the region's health manpower that could be released for national emergency service, the answers varied from about 10 to 40 percent, with an average of about 20 percent."

When asked what steps they would take to fill the gaps left by the departed physicians, Sigmond's respondents suggested a number of rearrangements, ranging from placing physician offices in hospitals (to reduce travel time) to making greater use of medical assistants.

But Sigmond's findings, like the findings of the presidential commission, do not bear out the validity of claims that there is a "shortage" of physicians.

"It seems clear that the 'shortage' of doctors and nurses is not
simply a matter of numbers but of efficiently utilizing the numbers
that now exist," Professor Glazer concluded.

Much of the insistence on a "doctor shortage" is based on a
week-long conference of medical educators in Fort Lauderdale,
Florida, in 1966. The Fort Lauderdale conference concluded that
the supply of physicians must be increased by at least four percent
per annum over the coming decade (or an increase from about
8,000 medical graduates a year to approximately 12,000 a year at
the end of the decade).

Eli Ginzberg of Columbia University, in his book *Men, Money &
Medicine*, discussed the considerations upon which the conferees
had based "this proposal for such a radical increase":

—the need to keep up with the rate of population increase;

—the need to compensate for physicians lost through retirement
or death;

—the need to keep up with increased demand resulting from
more spendable income *and government health programs*;

—increased time required by new procedures.

How valid are these considerations? It has been clearly illustrated
that the rate of increase in the physician population has been far
higher than merely keeping up with overall population increase or
normal physician attrition. It also seems distinctly ironic that advocates of national health insurance base claims of a health care crisis,
in part, on claims of a doctor shortage. They base claims of a doctor
shortage, in part, on *increased demand caused by government health
programs* and the need for more physician time with patients (the
very ingredient of health care that is most detrimentally affected by
the added burden of government regulations and paperwork requirements).

Claims of a "doctor shortage" rest on a flimsy foundation. For
example, Ginzberg lists among the other considerations that led to
the Fort Lauderdale conference's conclusions:

—the "desirability" of a better mix between young doctors and
old;

—a desire to replace foreign-born physicians on American hospital staffs with native physicians;

—a desire to create an abundance of physicians in the U.S. to encourage more American physicians to practice overseas in developing nations (to help create good will between the U.S. and developing nations);

—concern that the average American physician works too hard.

On such bases did the conference rest its insistence that the United States has a "doctor shortage"—a claim quickly picked up by the press and repeated by writers and politicians until it has become an almost unchallenged "fact." It has become a key part of the medical "crisis" campaign that national health insurance proponents hope to use to force a program through Congress in the coming months.

The truth is, the claims are based on whims, inaccurate figures, and unsubstantiated conclusions.

In determining the amount of physician increase needed to keep up with the population, for example, the conferees estimated that the population was increasing at the rate of 2 percent a year. According to the *Statistical Abstract of the U.S.,* issued by the Department of Commerce, the actual population growth at the time was 1.1 percent—and it later went down to 1.0 percent. In other words, projections based on the conference's assumptions were nearly 100 percent off at the time they were made.

There is absolutely no proof that an increase in spendable income increases demand for medical care—one of the assumptions adopted by the conferees. Ginzberg points out that the actual per capita income in the United States increased threefold between 1900 and 1960, far outpacing the increase in physicians. I have pointed out in Chapter 4 that the quality of the nation's health continued to improve at a rapid pace during that time. The point is made more clearly by the Bureau of Labor Statistics. According to the Bureau's figures for 1969 (see Chapter 5) the average "high-budget" family of four, with annual expenditures of approximately $11,000, spent only $26 a year more for health care than the "low-budget" family with annual expenditures of less than half as much.

Underlying the shrill insistence on the existence of a doctor shortage, and the impatient demands that something be done about it, is an assumption that the presence or absence of medical doctors is the prime determinant of the nation's health. That may not be so. Dr. Victor R. Fuchs, Professor of Economics and Community Medicine at the City University of New York, writing in the *New York Times* on December 19, 1970, pointed out that it is "extremely unlikely" that an increase in the number of physicians will have much impact on the health of the average American.

"Additional physicians could probably do little to reduce the heart attacks, lung cancer, alcoholism or motor accidents that destroy so many American men," Dr. Fuchs said. "Or consider the high infant mortality rates in the ghettos. Malnutrition, unwanted pregnancies, unsanitary home conditions and numerous other environmental and behavioral problems would result in unconscionably high infant death rates even if every pregnant woman received Park Avenue medical treatment."

There are other factors, too. For example, at least two major developments have combined to make the physician of today far more productive than his counterpart of a decade ago and earlier:

1. The trend toward specialization. As of the end of 1969, the old "family doctor" general practitioner of a few years ago had been so completely replaced by specialists that the GP accounted for only slightly more than one-fifth of the number of doctors involved in actual patient care.

According to the American Medical Association, of the 270,737 physicians seeing patients, only 57,845 were primarily in general practice—a smaller number than in any of the three specialty breakdowns (medical, surgical, miscellaneous). By contrast, there were 62,592 in medical specialties (internal medicine, dermatology, pediatrics, etc.); 79,005 in surgical specialties; and 71,295 in "other" specialties.

The trend toward specialization has had major effects on the nature of American medical care and has been widely criticized, both within the profession and without, for the depersonalization that results as more and more patients find themselves visiting doctors only for treatment of the specific illnesses (or surgical needs) within their domains.

In addition, the specialization of doctors reduces the number of doctors available for initial entry into the medical system, putting a heavy load on the relatively few general practitioners.

Because of these drawbacks, there has been a major effort in recent years to reverse the trend. The American Medical Association has created a new "specialty"—family practice—and several major medical colleges, most notably Penn State (at Hershey, Pa.) and the Medical College of South Carolina (at Charleston), have placed new emphasis on the development of family doctors.

Nonetheless, specialization has had one good effect: it has enabled each specialist, by developing expertise in one area of medicine, to perform more competently. There is less time wasted in experimentation and consultation. Many patients go directly to specialists such as internists, gynecologists, pediatricians and dermatologists, and thus bypass the cost and delay of being routed first through a referring general practitioner.

Clearly, specialization is neither an unmixed blessing nor an unmixed curse. But it does help to make today's physician more productive than yesterday's horse-and-buggy doctor.

2. Better use of the physician's time.

It is ironic that some patients—prodded by the cheerleading of medicine's critics—grumble about the fact that "doctors no longer make house calls." That, of course, is not completely true. Most doctors do make house calls on occasion, if the call is warranted, and some—especially those with a number of elderly patients—make large numbers of house calls.

Yet the house call, as a common medical practice, has gone by the wayside. During the period July, 1966, through June, 1967, only 3.4 percent of all physician visits with white patients took place inside the patient's home. The figure was even lower (2.2 percent) for non-white patients. But that trend—widely criticized though it is—is a sign of medical progress.

The family doctor of a few years ago was a highly mobile professional. Given a horse and buggy, or a car, and a good black bag, he could take his practice with him from home to home. His tools were limited and primitive; his pharmaceutical armamentarium was meager at best. In those days, thankfully gone by, the doctor's main assets—his education and his comforting "bedside manner"—were easily transportable from place to place.

Not so today. The modern physician's office is a storehouse of highly developed diagnostic and testing equipment. His office has become a miniature hospital, with X-rays, electrocardiograph machines, laboratory facilities. He is armed with vast supplies of lifesaving "miracle" drugs unknown a few decades ago.

The truth is, any doctor who routinely rushed to a patient's home with only the medical tools he could fit into a tiny black bag would be guilty, today, of first-rate medical incompetence—and probably would be rewarded with poor results. In the terms of the moderns, the office—or the hospital—is where the action is. Because it is where the help is.

In today's highly mobile society, a patient can reach the doctor's office, or a hospital, as quickly as the doctor can reach the patient. (It is no longer true that the doctor has one of the few autos in town.) The patient can thus be treated with the equipment and medicines made available by decades of technological and scientific advancement.

Today's doctor does not refrain from making house calls because he does not want to be bothered. Studies indicate that doctors voluntarily put in far more hours of work than the average layman, and frequently rush to perform hospital service, or meet patients at their offices, far into the evening (or early morning). Doctors insist that the patient come to the office simply because that is where the doctor can provide the highest degree of care.

More efficient use of office and hospital facilities, new medical equipment, and increased use of paramedical assistants have helped physicians increase productivity. Today, fewer doctors are needed to serve a given population. Despite these facts—despite the fact that health industry manpower increased by 90 percent during the 50s and early 60s—the cry continues: "There are not enough doctors; we must have more."

President Nixon, in his national health proposal, has suggested a system of Federal grants to medical schools based on the number of students graduated—an obvious incentive to step up greatly the output of doctors. There have been other calls for a greatly increased number of medical graduates. Loud voices urge more medical schools, bigger classes, more doctors. Yet that is a road that must be followed with caution.

There were far more medical schools in the United States at the turn of this century than there are today. In 1900, there were approximately 200; by 1930, the figure had been reduced to 76, with only 21,982 students and 4,735 graduates. By the 1969–70 school year, there were still only 101 schools—half as many as in

1900—with 37, 669 students and 8,367 graduates. But the decline was intentional, and the result was beneficial.

Michael Michaelson, editor of *ITIS*, a journal of health affairs for the city of Philadelphia, has written—accurately—that, "Until the turn of the twentieth century, American doctors were characteristically the products of 200 shoddy diploma mills . . ." Abraham Flexner, in his famous 1910 report on "Medical Education in the United States and Canada," characterized the medical teachers of the day as "loose and shifting bands of practicing physicians, calling themselves a faculty."

Flexner's report had a major impact on medical education, causing a number of medical schools to be closed. Medical education, and consequently patient care, have suffered to some extent as a result of Flexner's campaign. For example, in striving to improve the caliber of medical faculty, schools soon replaced all, or almost all, part-time faculty (usually active practitioners) with full-time salaried teachers. The result was a slow weaning of students from appreciation of patient care, and a substantial increase in the number of new doctors going into such duties as research, administration and teaching. Too, the number of medical graduates was substantially reduced. But the Flexner report had one good result: it wiped out the "shoddy diploma mill." Today's doctor is a graduate of a top-rate medical college, with high standards and rigorous requirements for graduation.

The current tendency to "open up" the medical schools will be both good and bad.

Some of the beneficiaries of this "opening up" will be academically qualified students—black, white or whatever—who have shown the aptitude to learn the exacting science and delicate art of practicing medicine, but who are unable to meet the ever-increasing costs of higher education. Tuition grants and scholarships can be a big help in opening the doors to a medical education for many young men and women with financial problems.

But many of the loudest cries for expanding the numbers of medical graduates come from those who would "open the doors" to minority group members, irrespective of scholastic qualification —who would not only lubricate the gates of admission, but also drop the academic bars that serve to weed out those who have shown an inability to comprehend, an unwillingness to work, a tendency to be easily diverted, or whatever else leads to lower than superior grades.

It is argued that stiff academic requirements create a "de facto discrimination"—that is, members of minority groups tend to be weeded out by collegiate grade-average standards (an academic poll tax), and that reliance on such superficial admission requirements is discriminatory and holds down the number of graduated doctors.

From the standpoint of the patient, it is not really relevant whether members of minority groups are or are not more frequently found in lower or higher scholastic ranges. All that is relevant to the patient is the competence of the final product: the practicing physician. When a patient is taken ill, his recovery depends in large part on the skill, intelligence, dedication, singlemindedness and integrity of his physician. It will be little solace to the patient who is wrongly treated to know that he has helped to achieve racial balance, or has been worked on by a doctor who was graduated to help fill an assumed "number of doctors" gap.

To those who argue that we will be turning out more doctors to serve in the areas where minority groups congregate, is it not discrimination against the residents of those areas to send them doctors who were admitted and passed from medical school on a basis of racial balance or the "need for more doctors" rather than competence? Is it not discrimination to give these poor people doctors who are not qualified to practice top-quality medicine?

That is what will be likely to happen.

Once a medical student is admitted, the die will be cast. The chances are very slim that those who chose to admit him on a basis of lower standards are subsequently going to flunk him if he does not keep up with the 3.8- or 3.9-average students in his class. If they do, they will (1) be admitting failure, (2) be laying themselves open to criticism they were only putting on a show of non-discrimination (because a bigger percentage of this "open-door" group will naturally be failed in proportion to the whole) and (3) be forfeiting cash grants based on numbers of graduates. So, with lower standards they will be admitted; with lower standards they will be graduated; with lower standards they will practice.

The victim of it all will be, ultimately, the patient.

There are, of course, ways to increase the number of medical graduates without decreasing the quality of doctors in the market-place. For example: construction of new, rigidly supervised medical schools; reassignment of facilities to provide more classroom space, and greater use of qualified practitioners as part-time faculty. There are even ways to ensure that more of the students admitted and graduated are members of minority groups—by using private, corporate, and charitable scholarships to ease financial burdens; making available competent tutoring for students with inadequate education but sufficient intelligence; and promoting the idea of health careers among minority-group students in junior and senior high schools.

It is not at all impossible to increase the number of medical graduates in the United States. Yet one must be very cautious about buying the wares of the "crisis" hawkers who urge major changes "now," including immediate increases in class sizes and immediate enrollment of students who would not now qualify for admission to medical schools. It would be disastrous to follow the desire for more doctors into a return to the "shoddy diploma mills" of yesterday, with all of the serious consequences for the nation's patients.

To some extent, the so-called "doctor shortage" might be more aptly termed a "crisis of availability," since the essential criticisms are often based on (a) the number of doctors performing services of patient care, and (b) the availability of doctors and other health care facilities to the average citizen.

Ironically, 11 months after *Medical News Report* wrote of the "health manpower shortage," the same publication reported that the number of full-time faculty in U.S. medical schools had increased twice as fast as the increase in medical students during the previous six years. At the beginning of 1971, there were 37,669 students and nearly 25,000 teachers. Therein lies part of the "availability" problem. Lured principally by Federal financial inducements, more and more physicians are entering such realms as research, teaching, administrative work and planning. Large bodies of doctors, working for various governments or supported by government grants, never treat a patient.

At the end of 1969, there were 28,000 MDs in government service—more than in nearly half the states combined. Some 6,000 doctors—enough to staff a city the size of Chicago; nearly 2.5 times as many as practice in the state of Oklahoma—work for the Federal Government in jobs in which they provide no patient care. National health insurance will simply increase the problem. More government medicine will mean more administration, more planning—and more doctors not taking care of patient needs.

Critics frequently contend that American physicians are poorly distributed throughout the nation, with noticeable gaps in rural areas and the older sections of major cities. This alleged maldistribution is one of the problems they propose to cure with national health insurance.

Clearly there are areas in which the supply of medical manpower is limited. Unfortunately, it will take more than a system change to cure some of those problems. Doctors practicing in burned-out, crime-ridden sections of large cities are eager to leave. It will not be easy to find others to take their place. Doctors who seek cultural advantages such as opera houses and symphony halls—or even doctors who want only a choice of movies—will hesitate to move to rural areas far distant from large cities. Persons who choose to live in the quiet atmosphere of rural America must pay a price for it—the price of forgoing the services of persons who might not share a desire for the same style of life.

There will, of course, always be some doctors who will practice in the inner city, and others who will practice in rural communities, either because they enjoy the life style or because they are responding to altruistic instincts. But there will probably always be a lesser number of doctors in those areas than in the comfortable suburbs. Nor is national health insurance likely to change that situation except through compulsion. The limited financial incentives under government medical programs simply will not lure most physicians into undesirable life situations.

The truth is, most Americans have ready access to medical treatment. Dr. Morris Fishbein, the highly respected editor of *Medical World News*, has pointed out that, "While there are slum areas with only one or two doctors to care for many thousands of people, at close hand are the medical services of such great hospitals as Johns Hopkins, New York Hospital and literally a thousand others."

Dr. Fishbein's analysis was documented by the 1967 report of the presidential Commission on Health Manpower: ". . . physical distance from available care is not a major barrier for either urban or rural residents," the Commission reported. "Even in rural areas, hospital facilities of 25 beds or more are within a 25-mile distance of all but 2 percent of the population, and only one-tenth of one percent have to travel more than 50 miles. Home-to-work commuting patterns of rural populations suggest that an hour's drive is not prohibitive for such routine purposes as shopping and entertainment, much less for the infrequent visits which might be needed for health care. In the urban areas, none of the population is more than 10 miles from a hospital."

The "maldistribution crisis," like the "doctor shortage" itself, is a myth. While there is always room for improvement—and always a desire for more doctors, closer—it seems clear that both in terms of numbers and distribution, the cries of a "doctor shortage" are made up more of rhetoric than of reality.

7. The Non-System

The campaign for national health insurance rests on a base of catchphrases and slogans. Of these, none is repeated more fervently than the charge that the American medical system is not really one at all; that it is a "non-system."

Fortune magazine calls American medicine a "cottage industry."

Daniel Schorr, in his book *Don't Get Sick in America*, writes of "Corner Grocery" hospitals and "Pushcart Peddler" doctors.

"The fact is," states the Committee for National Health Insurance, "we do not have a health-care system at all. We have a non-system."

Barbara and John Ehrenreich, co-authors of *The American Health Empire*, sum up the common diagnosis of such liberals as New York's Mayor John Lindsay, labor leaders Harold Gibbons (of the Teamsters) and the late Walter Reuther, civil rights leaders such as Mrs. Martin Luther King, Jr., and the late Whitney Young, Jr. ". . . medical care is simply adrift," they say. "It is dominated by small, inefficient and uncoordinated enterprises (private doctors, small hospitals, and nursing homes), which add up to a fragmented and wasteful whole—a non-system." The Ehrenreichs, whose vitriolic book condemns the medical profession in broad denunciations, without benefit of even a single substantiating footnote, disagree that America has no medical system. It is a non-system only in terms of providing care, they say; it is very much a system in terms of its primary goal, which they say is the business of making a profit.

The planners are so perturbed by the non-system they purport to find, so passionate and repetitious in their insistences, that even such a fully accredited liberal as Dr. Alex Gerber, an advocate of national health insurance, has been forced to put things back in perspective: "They tell us that we are a 'cottage industry' doing anachronistic 'piecework,' as though medical care were comparable to sewing buttons on a coat in a factory," he writes. "The derisive epithet 'nonsystem of health care'—or better, 'an outmoded, Model T, nonsystem'—has been abused until it abrades the ear with rivet-hammer effect."

Is there a health-care "system" in the United States? In the terms envisioned by the planners, there fortunately is not.

The American health-care "system," such as it is, is simple, relatively inexpensive, and efficient. And it preserves the freedoms and privacy of both patient and doctor.

Simply put, the American health-care system operates like this:

A patient goes to whatever physician he chooses—a general practitioner or, if the patient has isolated the problem, directly to a specialist. If the general practitioner is unable to deal with the specifics of the illness, *he* may send the patient to a specialist.

The patient is either treated in the office, or placed in a hospital. He may be directed to buy a medicine, or not.

After treatment, he is sent to his home or, if a lengthier supervised recuperation is required, to a convalescence facility.

For most Americans, the method of payment is equally simple: they select a personal physician and pay him whenever they use his services; if the doctor writes a prescription, the patient pays the pharmacist for the capsules or mixtures he provides; if the patient is hospitalized, he pays for the treatment he receives and the days he spends in the hospital. The bills are paid either by the patient or by a private third party, usually an insurance company.

Under this system of private practice, the patient pays only for the care or service he receives. If he receives 20 minutes of a physician's time, that is what he pays for, regardless of how much service the physician renders to the other patients he sees that day. The customer in a drug store pays only for the number of pills he is given without concern for how many pills the druggist's other customers are purchasing. The patient pays only for his own time in a hospital, plus his pro rata share of the hospital's overhead; he does not pay for the time spent by the other patients.

As a general rule, none of the participants in the health-care process will be closely associated with another. Each stop along the way—the general practitioner, the specialist, the pharmacist, the hospital, the convalescence facility—is a separate service, operated by individuals or groups of individuals.

The system is simple (one step logically follows another), it is efficient (each step may be the last in the process, unless further steps are required), it is fair (at each step in the process, the patient can elect to go further or not, to follow the doctor's directions or ignore them, to remain with the physician or go to another, to buy medicine from one pharmacy or another, to use one hospital or another).

Unfortunately, this system of private enterprise medicine is so familiar to most of us that we seldom stop to marvel at its classic simplicity. Yet, despite its simplicity, it *is* a system—and a system that has worked to provide high quality health care to the American people at a reasonable cost. In its place, advocates of government medicine would erect a complex, impersonal, highly structured— and highly expensive—system of mass medical treatment.

The simplicity of the American medical system drives social planners up the wall; the delivery of health care, like daily activity in all phases of personal and public life, is considered inefficient unless supervised by central bureaus of overseers and guided by carefully delineated regulations. Complexity, not simplicity, is the hallmark of governmental planning.

Planning has become a fetish for those who advocate new government takeovers. Operating from an assumption of bureaucratic or legislative omniscience (that is, assuming that all brains are in Washington), the planners righteously insist on a corresponding omnipotence in one area after another. After all, what good does it do to know what is good for Harry, better than he himself knows it, if one is not empowered to bring about the results?

This unbelievable arrogance is central to the concept of Federal planning, and central, therefore, to the insistent cries for a more complex, more rigidly structured, "system" of medical care—a system in which Federal legislators and administrators will determine what fees for service are proper and what fees are not; what duration of hospitalization is required for a particular illness; what medication and what treatment are best suited for a patient whose medical history is unknown to the planner.

Already, even without national health insurance, there is an increasing tendency for lawmakers and law-administrators to appropriate to themselves the responsibilities of health care. Under the aegis of Medicare and Medicaid, bureaucrats have undertaken to supervise medical treatment through the ultimate weapon available to them: the ability to withhold payment for service. In every community, physicians have been subjected to bureaucratic questioning in connection with claims for treatment rendered under Federal programs. Following type-bound guidelines, without ever seeing the patient for whom the services were rendered, non-physicians working for payment intermediaries challenge treatments rendered, medication prescribed, number of visits by the patient to a doctor's office, or by the doctor to a patient's home or hospital room.

Many a general practitioner can tell of the patient whose symptoms defied classification, who failed to react to standard clinical treatment, but who responded immediately (and mysteriously) to vitamin injections, placebos or other non-standard modes of care. For these reasons—because medicine is still an art as well as a science; because the doctor deals with individual people, with psychological and physiological differences and different psychological and physiological needs—doctors insist they must not be hampered by rigid regulations that would bureaucratically establish "approved" treatments.

Unfortunately, as bureaucracy proliferates, the tendency to plan by rote becomes greater. Patients are put in a mold, and individual eccentricities—both psychological and physiological—are ignored. Patients become statistics. In fact, much of this attitude is evident in the current popularity of the terms "provider" and "consumer" —computerized abstractions for the real people we used to know as doctors and patients, or as Doc Harry Wilson at the corner of Elm and Grove, and old Mrs. Thompson, who has a bad pain in her back every so often for which medicine can find no explanation, but which Doctor Wilson has learned to cure over the years. There is no room in a "system" for Doc Wilson, Mrs. Thompson, or the "miracle" unapproved cure for an insufficiently diagnosed back ailment.

It seems axiomatic, however, that highly structured systems are not essential to all forms of endeavor; in fact, it is readily apparent that there are many relationships that function more satisfactorily in a less rigid format. While supermarkets may bring wider varieties of food, at quantity prices, to more people, the supermarket concept may be totally unsuited for the provision of services that require individual attention rather than rolling baskets and check-out lines. Clearly, for example, the "cottage industry" or "non-system" —the personal one-to-one confrontation—is a more satisfactory method of handling the relationship between the confessor and his priest, the lawyer and his client, the husband and his wife. I submit the same is true of the intimate and highly personal relationship between a patient and his or her doctor.

Dr. Michael J. Halberstam, a self-professed medical liberal, answered critics of the "non-system" in a 1969 speech in Chicago. "Of course, medicine is primarily a cottage industry," he said, "depending as it usually does on the mutual respect and trust of two individuals, the one seeking help, the other giving it. Medicine starts in that cry for help, and ultimately comes back to it. Medicine can be practiced on the assembly line, but I doubt if we want it."

Fortunately, Americans still have an opportunity to choose. Patients in other nations are not so fortunate. For them, assembly-line medicine is a painful fact. When British reporter Joan Hobson approached a patient coming out of a Nottinghamshire Health Centre, he looked at her, then back at the health center, and said simply, "I feel like I've been processed."

Mrs. Hobson found the same reaction throughout Britain's highly systematized network of health-care facilities. "When I get here there's no guarantee I shall see my own doctor," a white-haired lady complained at a center in Bedfordshire. "I find the place very impersonal . . ." Another woman whispered: "Previously I knew that my doctor would visit when I needed him, but now it could be any of the doctors who work here. In five consultations I haven't seen the same man twice."

Each health-center patient does get to select a personal doctor from among the clinic staff, but there is no assurance that the chosen doctor will be the one to come through the door. As a result, British patients no longer enjoy the rapport with their physicians that Americans have come to rely upon.

One man, waiting in a center near Brighton, complained about the loss of the personal relationships. "I know that doctors are busy people," he said, "and it is not likely that my doctor remembered *me* in great detail, but at least I knew *him,* and as each interview progressed the rapport we had earlier established was renewed and developed. Now it's often a fellow I've never met previously and unless I ask him directly, or can make out the signature on his prescription, I don't even get to know with whom I've been discussing intimate aspects of my life. I feel like a case history rather than an individual."

Not only do patients under government systems lose their individual identities, they also lose their human identities. For example, a new health center in Sussex has developed a system within the system: as patients are ushered into the large waiting room, they are directed to rows of colored chairs: patients who are scheduled to see Dr. X are seated on red chairs; patients to see Dr. Y are guided to green chairs. Patients are summoned to numbered consulting rooms by means of a loudspeaker.

Mrs. Hobson had an opportunity to undergo treatment in the system herself when she injured a foot and entered a 12-doctor health center. She described the incident in an article in *Private Practice.* "I was instructed to pass down an orange-linoleumed corridor until I reached a mauve door," she said. "On the way I met a man who remarked, 'We're like a lot of ants following trails so that scientists can use us for study. They'll be putting us on conveyor belts next.' "

But it is not the doctors who are "using" the patients. They, too, are victims of the system and they, too, bemoan the loss of rapport with the individuals they must attempt to heal.

"Patients are becoming mere ciphers," complains Dr. Paul Sharpe. "Registration numbers, identification digits and NHS numbers now figure so much in my work that I sometimes feel more like a mathematician than a physician."

Meanwhile, the centers grow larger and more impersonal. Several new centers planned for Glasgow will each house 25 practitioners. A health center currently under construction in Middlesborough will house 21 doctors, responsible for 62,000 patients. "A proper personal service just cannot be given in this way," a Newcastle doctor complained recently.

But depersonalization is part of the price one must pay for a system of the sort envisioned by the planners. Depersonalization—in fact, dehumanization—flows directly from the assembly-line techniques of the systematists.

Impersonal experience with mass medicine is not limited to the patients in Surrey or physicians in Newcastle. Many Americans have been exposed to similar treatment in the large pre-payment facilities in some of our major cities. One of the first of these, which often serves as a model for the planners, was the large Kaiser Permanente facility in California. Dr. G. H. Hoehn, of San Gabriel, recently described some of his experiences with patients who had come to his offices after unpleasant encounters with the mass-treatment approach at Kaiser. "Many of us have patients who pay hard-earned money for private care even though they are eligible for 'free' care by closed-panel groups [pre-payment clinics in which patients are treated by a staff of salaried physicians], and this at a time when so many are complaining about medical fees," Dr. Hoehn said. "What motivates these people to pay for what they could be getting free? The advertising geniuses say the word 'free' has the most powerful appeal in the world. These patients must have even more powerful reasons for choosing to *pay* for their care."

Dr. Hoehn then proceeded to detail some actual case histories that shed some light on the decisions.

—J.C., a 50-year-old working man suffering from a painful rash, came to Dr. Hoehn after first trying Kaiser Permanente. At Kaiser, complained the patient, after a long wait marked by the completion of burdensome forms and questionnaires, he had been admitted to the presence of a busy dermatologist who took a quick look at the rash, prescribed a steroid ointment, and walked out.

The Kaiser specialist—highly trained and board certified—had apparently been unable to take the time to quiz J.C. about his work or hobbies to see what might be causing the rash, even though such routine questioning is standard procedure for most dermatologists. The doctor offered no advice on hand care to avoid recurrence of the rash, and did not prescribe any of the internal antihistamines that would have eased the annoying itch that kept the patient awake at night.

After the rash had persisted for three more months, the patient, in desperation, called on Dr. Hoehn. J.C. complained that he had been sloughed off, that he left the Kaiser doctor's examining room with an annoying feeling that his unspectacular rash had simply bored the specialist who had examined him. Dr. Hoehn proceeded to clear up the rash "almost immediately."

Dr. Hoehn is probably not any more qualified at his work than is the Kaiser doctor, and does not claim to be. But in the private doctor's office the patient had received one vital ingredient that had been missing at the Kaiser assembly line: personal attention.

First, Dr. Hoehn took the time to quiz J.C. about the soaps and chemicals he used, and then gave him instructions on hand care. Noticing that the skin had thickened in the area of the rash—a natural reaction by which the body attempts to protect itself—Dr. Hoehn treated his patient with Grenz ray to reduce the thickening and, because the thick protective covering prevented absorption of the medicated ointment, he prescribed that the steroid be given by injection instead. Learning that J.C. had been having trouble sleeping, Dr. Hoehn prescribed antihistamines to ease the itching.

If the Kaiser doctor's care had been routine, so had Dr. Hoehn's. If Dr. Hoehn's treatment had been in accord with quality medical practice, so had that of the Kaiser doctor. The simple difference was the extra attention—the *personal* attention—Dr. Hoehn had given his patient. At Kaiser, the patient was a rash; in Dr. Hoehn's office, the patient was J.C., a middle-aged working man with specific exposures to rash-causing chemicals and difficulty in sleeping.

The Kaiser treatment cost J.C. nothing; his employer had pre-paid for his medical care at the year's start. Dr. Hoehn's attention and treatment cost him $20. But J.C. reported immediate relief after the private care and three months of continued rash after treatment by the "system."

—Mrs. M.A. had received sound advice from Kaiser dermatologists but was getting nowhere in attempting to heal her dermatitis. Under Dr. Hoehn's attention, she had rapid progress and the problem soon disappeared.

Again, Dr. Hoehn was no better a doctor than the qualified men at the "system" facility. The difference was: each time "the patient" returned to Kaiser she was seen by a different doctor and thus received different orders and different advice, sometimes contradicting the orders and advice she had received earlier. Although there is usually more than one effective regimen for treatment, she was not being maintained on any one program of care, but was instead "starting over" with each visit and each new doctor.

It was not Dr. Hoehn who cured Mrs. M.A.: it was the simple fact that she was following a consistent treatment because Dr. Hoehn—and *only* Dr. Hoehn—was her doctor.

—E.B.'s case is best told in Dr. Hoehn's own words:

"Little E.B.'s mother left (Kaiser) because of a mountain of little complaints: too crowded, a feeling of being herded through, no personal attention, too far to travel, frequent visits with very little accomplished (I saw him only once a month), changeover of doctors and nurses and receptionists, and a little child's fear of strangers. In our office he felt at home with the nurses by the third visit. They knew his first name by then and he felt secure because he had found we aren't 'shot happy' when it comes to little children. E.B.'s parents are in a low-income group, but the mother feels our care is worth it."

Dr. Hoehn's report appeared in *Private Practice*, a medical journal read only by physicians. This was no attempt by him to demonstrate his exceptional abilities, for his patients would never see the report. Besides, he claims no exceptional talents other than the one that is shared by the nearly 200,000 physicians who offer private, fee-for-service medical care: personal treatment.

The situations presented by these patients are really the same, Dr. Hoehn says. "The problem is: Who is the doctor working for? Who is his master? It is still axiomatic that we can have only one master. Either we are working for the patient and have his interest foremost, or we are working for Kaiser . . . When a closed panel (pre-payment group) is the employer, and is getting a limited amount for each patient, there is bound to be underuse of the facility—money is saved at the patient's expense."

The system, as Dr. Hoehn discovered through the reports of his patients, contains a number of drawbacks. Among them:

—A tendency by doctors to reduce overhead by proffering minimal care, although always within the guidelines of sound medical treatment. The danger, of course, is that sound care "by the book" may not be sufficient, as it was not in the case of J.C.'s rash. It is people, not rashes or diseases, who come to physicians for help, and proper care may require more than cursory examination and perfunctory treatments.

—A tendency for doctors to become lackadaisical and bored by repeated exposure to unspectacular cases. While the incentive of increased income through a growing reputation is usually enough to overcome this tendency among private practitioners, there is no such incentive among physicians in pre-payment groups who are paid fixed salaries.

—Physicians in private practice frequently build up competent and experienced office staffs, capable of prompt and efficient execution of the physician's orders. In large facilities, with correspondingly large staffs and frequent turnover, physicians may find themselves forced to spend more time simply explaining instructions, writing prescriptions or often performing "utilitarian services"—time that thus becomes unavailable for direct patient care.

—Constant shuffling of patients from doctor to doctor increases the time each physician must spend, on each visit, if he is to provide optimum care. Each time the patient visits the facility, the new doctor on the assignment must decipher his predecessor's notes that, even in normal detail, insufficiently explain *why* a doctor followed a certain course of treatment. Thus, each doctor must routinely approve earlier treatment, without fully understanding the reason for it, or simply start over, with the resultant contradictory orders and advice that drove Mrs. M.A. to Dr. Hoehn's office.

To planners who suggest that mass pre-payment centers can be made to be friendly and personal, Dr. Hoehn replies: "You simply can't transform a big impersonal giant into a warm, friendly individual."

He is right, of course. The choices are between the impersonal system or the personal non-system.

If one seeks a rigidly structured system "for utmost efficiency," one must be prepared to accept the assembly-line techniques and depersonalization that flow from it. And, ironically, because rigid systems reduce incentive, eliminate opportunity for innovation, and place decision-making powers in inflexible guidebooks, one must also be prepared to accept the *decrease* in efficiency that inevitably follows every attempt to adapt mass-production manufacturing techniques to personal services.

The planners insist on the right to adopt contradictions simultaneously. For example, they insist on centralized planning to reduce "wasteful duplication" by limiting expensive and infrequently used equipment to one or two central facilities, and simultaneously complain of maldistribution if segments of the population must travel long distances to reach such care. This petulant insistence, couched in terms of scientific and philosophic intellectualism, boils down simply to a *demand* that one be able to eat his cake and have it too.

So it is with those who simultaneously (1) call for the creation of a highly structured system, and (2) demand the retention of those qualities—personal attention, more time spent with patients, progressive care—that flourish only in the atmosphere of the individualized non-system they decry.

A young radical took the microphone at the American Medical Association's 1970 convention in Chicago and insisted that the non-system be replaced with a system; that physicians turn over more of their patient care to paramedics (auxiliary medical personnel); that doctors, in short become more efficient. In the same statement, the same speaker complained bitterly that physicians spend too little time with their patients. He complained that his own physician refused to take the time to sip a cup of coffee with him and discuss his ailments at greater length, in a more personal manner!

This young radical, typical of the group that has branded the AMA an "American Murder Association," was echoing a common unwillingness to accept reality. What he was saying, in effect, was "I want something to be both A and non-A at the same time; why can't it be both something and something else at the same time? Don't you understand? I *insist* that it be both A and non-A at the same time; I *demand* it."

Unfortunately, just as the advocates of free enterprise medicine must accept that system for both its virtues and its failings—trying always to maximize the one and minimize the other—the advocates of the new "system" must be prepared to accept the concept for what it offers and what it fails to offer. And personal care is not one of the things available on an assembly line.

Dr. Hoehn, of course, is a private practitioner. One might reasonably ask, then, if his criticisms are exaggerated and influenced by the fact that, due to the insistence of the planners, the pre-payment facilities he attacks are a direct threat to the continued existence of his type of medical practice. But private, fee-for-service practitioners are not the only doctors who have publicly noted the major drawbacks to highly systematized medical care in mass-pre-payment facilities.

Dr. Sidney Garfield, a long-time promoter of the pre-payment group approach to medicine and a founder of Kaiser Permanente, is candid about the disadvantages of such a system. "Pre-payment makes medical care a right by eliminating fee-for-service, and for years we have been deeply concerned with our relative inability to keep up with the soaring demand that this right produces, and to maintain a level of service satisfactory to us," Dr. Garfield admitted in a 1970 speech to the American Association of Public Health Physicians.

"It is distressing to realize that elimination of fees can be as much a barrier to early care as the fee itself," he said. "The reason is that when we removed the fee, we removed the regulator of flow into the system. The result is a massive uncontrolled flood of . . . the well, the worried well, the early sick and the sick, into the point of entry—the doctor's appointment—on a first-come-first-served basis that has little relation to priority of need. The impact of this demand overloads the system and, since the well and worried well are a large component of that entry mix, their usurping of doctor time actually acts as a barrier to the entry of the sick.

"The same thing is happening to medical care throughout the country. The traditional delivery system, which has evolved under fee-for-service, is being overwhelmed because of the elimination of personally paid fees through the spread of health insurance, Medi-care and Medicaid. This floods the system not only with increased numbers of people but with . . . a large proportion of relatively well people."

Dr. Garfield's proposed solution was a further decrease in the personal nature of medical care—a computerized health testing procedure, manned by medical assistants, which would be used to ration the number of patients permitted actually to discuss their ailments, real or imagined, with a doctor.

The surrender of personal care, a corollary to structured health-care systems, may, as in Dr. Garfield's proposal, be increased, rather than reduced, as operators of the system seek means to solve the other problems inherent in "free" government medicine: political determination of financial priorities, centralization of facilities, and, as in the case at Kaiser, soaring public demand for what patients believe to be "free" care. Clearly, the failures of the system feed upon themselves, each leading to a further deterioration of care as non-medical problems become paramount and physicians, rather than worrying about new healings for patient illnesses, find themselves increasingly concerned with such problems as regulation of the demands upon their time, or talking the system's managers out of enough funds for necessary equipment and facilities.

Dr. Garfield, who has helped to create a medical "system," and who now is trying to make it work efficiently, concedes that the problems he now faces are in the nature of government-financed medical care:

"The delivery system functioned fairly well with fee-for-service under which it evolved," he says. "It became unbalanced and a so-called 'non-system' under the impact of the poorly planned legislation of Medicare and Medicaid with its elimination of fees, and that result should not surprise anyone. Picture what would happen to air transportation if fares were eliminated and travel became a right. What chance would you have of getting anyplace if you really needed to? Even the highly automated telephone service would be staggered by removal of fees and necessary calls would become practically impossible. The change from 'fee' to 'free' would disrupt any system in the country no matter how well organized, and this is particularly true of medicine with its highly personalized sick-care service.

"National health insurance," Dr. Garfield cautions, "will only make matters worse."

Despite such warnings, however, the push for a new system continues, primarily in the Kennedy and Nixon health programs. The Kennedy plan would allocate a portion of the income from national health insurance taxation to development of group prepayment plans, under official government sponsorship. Although private practice would be permitted, the payment schedules would be strongly weighted to discourage such a manner of practice. For example, under the Kennedy plan, all prescribed drugs would be covered in full by the plan's benefits if prescribed by a doctor in a group pre-payment plan, but only maintenance drugs would be covered if prescribed by a private physician practicing by the more personalized traditional fee-for-service method. Obviously, a patient expecting to receive a pharmaceutical prescription would be inclined to visit a group doctor rather than pay a second time for the medicine (having paid for it once through taxation).

The group plan concept is further promoted by the payment provision of the law. Benefits would be paid first to institutional providers of care (including hospitals and clinics) and then to pre-payment group practices and fee-for-service practitioners. Pre-payment group physicians and fee-for-service physicians would be paid a proportionate share of their fees, *based on comprehensiveness of service.* Thus, a large group would receive a larger percentage of its bill for each patient than would an individual physician. Obviously, such a program will effectively force many physicians into large group plans or out of practice entirely.

Nixon's health plan, though less extensive, would also attempt to force patients into a new Federally ordained "system," with government loans and grants to be used to encourage the formation of "health maintenance organizations" (the administration's new description of pre-payment plans). Administration spokesmen have stated that by the end of this decade they intend to have 90 percent of the American population treated by such large mass-care facilities rather than by their individual family physicians.

Backers of the Kennedy and Nixon plans defend their push for such impersonal assembly-line systems on the basis of the supposed need to develop some new means of controlling costs. The evidence indicates that mass "systems" have just the opposite effect. Dr. Edward S. Hyman, a New Orleans internist, discussed the cost effects of such medical systems in Senate testimony on behalf of the American Association of Councils of Medical Staffs, of which he is Secretary:

"Concerning the efficiency of our private 'non-system' versus Federal and state medicine," Dr. Hyman said, "The CMS calls your attention to the following data . . . [Dr. Hyman here projected a chart indicating per diem and total-stay costs for New Orleans area hospitals]. Note that in 1968 the private hospitals ranged from $392 to $648 per stay. Note that Charity Hospital, run by the state of Louisiana, was as expensive as the most expensive private hospitals, yet Charity Hospital claims a desperate and perennial deficit. Furthermore, the two Federal hospitals were *50 percent more expensive,* because the length of stay in government-run hospitals is that much longer. . . . Even minor cases stay long periods before final treatment or surgery.

"The CMS notes that whenever Federal controls were added to the hospital system, the hospital costs increased," he concluded.

Herbert E. Klarman, Professor of Environmental Medicine and Community Health at the State University of New York, has also expressed doubts about the ability of mass-pre-payment systems to deliver care less expensively or more efficiently. Speaking at the first International Congress on Group Practice, in 1970, Klarman said that although most of the interest in pre-paid group practice in the U.S. has been inspired by the hopes that the technique can cut health costs, several studies have cast doubt on the validity of such a conclusion. He pointed to a study of group practice in San Francisco, which found that as the size of the group increased, there was a corresponding increase in the amount of ancillary services provided, but no increase in efficiency.

Not only is there no guaranteed *increase* in efficiency under such a system, but the results may be just the opposite. For example, William A. Glaser, Director of International and Comparative Research for Columbia University's Bureau of Applied Social Research, in a book entitled *Paying the Doctor: Systems of Remuneration and Their Effects*, concluded that under a capitation (fixed annual pre-payment) system, there is a tendency for doctors to neglect their patients because there are no financial incentives for more effort or better quality.

The truth, despite the planners' complexity complex, is that bigness isn't always tantamount to quality. In a copyrighted article in *Medical Economics* entitled "Do Big Groups Breed Second-Rate Medicine?" Dr. Thomas Gladner (the name is a psuedonym) described some of his impressions gleaned during three years in a large midwestern group practice. Among his criticisms:

—As an internist, he was not permitted to select the specialist to whom he would refer patients. Instead, the specialists were "selected" on a rotation basis by business-office clerks, a policy determined by business, rather than patient care, priorities.

—Older doctors invariably ended up on the management committee, and in charge of the various departments. As a result, energetic young doctors, versed in modern methods, were forced to practice according to "the way we've always done it."

—One patient complained of feeling more like a TV set in a repair shop than a patient. Dr. Gladner admits that he himself had become a medical mechanic, treating diseases rather than people.

In another article in *Medical Economics*, entitled "Private Practice Can Revolutionize Health Care," Dr. Elsie A. Giorgi, Associate Clinical Professor of Community Medicine at the University of California's College of Medicine in Irvine, argued that group practices do not improve efficiency to the degree their proponents claim. Group practices don't cost the patient noticeably less, Dr. Giorgi said, and are sometimes *more* expensive than private care by an individual doctor. While the system didn't solve the cost problem, it contributed new ones of its own. For example, Dr. Giorgi reported hearing patients "complain of long waits even for urgent appointments" at what she called "the large and increasingly depersonalized group clinics."

Advocates of a new "system" frequently claim that the assembly-line groups are more economical, citing statistics that indicate that patients under such systems undergo less surgery and spend fewer days in the hospital, which, they contend, proves that they are kept in better health by their visits to the pre-payment centers. Such economies may not be blessings for the patient, however, if *underuse* —practiced in the name of economy—deprives the patient of beneficial care.

Evidence of the deficiencies of mass medical systems continues to mount, and as it does, amazingly, the shrill cry for a "system" grows louder. "Pre-paid group practice, a health care financing scheme that never made it big in all the years it has been around, has suddenly become the hottest among numerous ideas for reshaping the U.S. health system," *Medical News Report* stated on March 29, 1971.

Among the indicators:

—leadership of the American Hospital Association has endorsed the pre-payment concept;

—the National Association of Blue Shield Plans is working toward development of pre-paid group programs;

—nearly one-third of the nation's Blue Cross plans are working toward affiliation with pre-paid plans, and staffs of two major pre-payment facilities, Kaiser Permanente (California) and the Health Insurance Plan of Greater New York, are training Blue Cross staffers for pre-payment group management roles;

—a number of large corporations and insurance companies have expressed interest in starting pre-payment facilities of their own.

The drive for a "system" rolls on, gaining in strength each month. Proponents of a medical restructuring seem to be ignoring the evidence before them, evidence that is ignored only at increased risk to the potential patients under such a system (meaning, all of us).

America *has* had experience with government medical systems. In February, 1971, Dr. Jesse Steinfeld, the U.S. Surgeon General, admitted:

"Eighty percent . . . of the budget of the Department of Health, Education and Welfare is related to the major Federal programs for the purchase of health care for the elderly and the poor through Medicare and Medicaid. Needless to say, we are not completely satisfied that we have obtained our full money's worth, but we are working on a number of programs . . . to improve that care and make it less expensive and more accessible."

Dr. Steinfeld's disappointment with the effects of a medical "system" should come as no surprise. Germany has long had such a system, and has had similar results. More than a decade ago, in 1960, Theodor Blank, Germany's Minister of Labor, said, "It is intolerable both for the patients and the dignity of the medical profession to see, annually, more than seven billion marks contributed to compulsory health insurance, and despite all this, sick persons are not adequately taken care of, and the waiting rooms of the doctors are so overcrowded they cannot give anyone proper medical attention."

Dr. Joseph Boyle, Chairman of the Congress of County Medical Societies, recently recalled a discussion with a colleague who returned from a tour of Yugoslavia with representatives of the American College of Cardiology. "It seems that under Yugoslavia's brand of socialized medicine, something akin to a sick call is held each morning and afternoon," Dr. Boyle wrote. "Long queues of people enter a large auditorium, file down to the front of the room, and pass single file before a panel consisting of the Yugoslav equivalent of social workers, registered nurses, assistant physicians and physicians."

During one such assembly-line sick call, Dr. Boyle related, a woman patient appeared complaining of a marked swelling of the right arm. The woman was immediately referred to a local hospital and scheduled for a large number of complex diagnostic studies. Several days later, she was still waiting for the tests, with her right arm badly swollen. One of the American doctors asked permission to examine the woman. As soon as permission was granted, he removed the woman's gown—and discovered a tightly wound roll of bandage, secured by a tight band. The band and bandages were removed and the swelling disappeared.

Such is the danger of the mass-care system that treats symptoms and illnesses, rather than people; that herds patients past assembly-line stations of cursory, impersonal care.

Dr. Russell Roth, speaker of the AMA's House of Delegates, had an opportunity to observe a highly structured health-care system during a recent tour of the Soviet Union. In many ways, including the organization of care into large centralized facilities, the Soviet system is similar to systems that have been proposed as replacements for the "non-system" of medical care in the United States.

Although the Soviet system has its good points—most notably in mobile emergency care—it has a number of drawbacks as well. Soviet citizens are assigned to physicians and health-care facilities. Children are assigned to pediatricians and dentists; mothers to obstetrician-gynecologists and the area hospital; the husband, if he works at a major factory, will get his primary care there and will probably be hospitalized at the plant hospital; grandfather, who is retired, will be treated by the assigned physician for the area and at an assigned hospital. There is no free choice of physician, and no free choice of hospital.

"The vast majority of physicians practicing in Russia today have been educated in didactic vocational schools designed to try to make of them competent technicians practicing medicine by the book . . . ," Dr. Roth reported. "There are mandated ways of carrying out diagnosis and treatment, with little individualization. The whole authoritarian system is permeated with a feeling that patients must be satisfied with what they get, since the care is costing them nothing and they have no particular rights. Physicians follow the rules as laid down in the books or imposed by their superiors and tend to be preoccupied with the complexities of getting better pay and better assignments. . . .

"Americans, with some militance, proclaim their rights to personalized, high quality, competent care. The Russian, if he feels that he is endowed with such rights, usually knows better than to express the thought publicly."

Recognition of the failure of structured medical systems is implicit in one of the major criticisms leveled at the current non-system. Those who cry of a gap between the high quality of care received by the rich and the allegedly poor quality of care received by the poor, ignore the fact that it is *government* that shoulders the credit or the blame for the care the poor now receive. Whereas private doctors once voluntarily donated their care to the needy, that care has become increasingly the domain of the government —at the government's own insistence.

The poor, once treated charitably to the same care received by their more affluent neighbors, have been herded into municipal hospitals that are now universally condemned as archaic, dirty and inefficient. (An article in *Look* magazine, in May, 1971, described the horrible state of Chicago's Cook County Hospital, a prime example of government's failure to provide adequate medical care.) The poor, the veterans, the American Indian—all have been the subject of widespread public concern as evidence mounts of the poor quality of medical care available to them. Yet *none* of these groups are cared for by the private medical system—not because the doctors in that system are unwilling to provide the care, but because the responsibility has been pre-empted by government. The failure to provide good health care to the poor rests on the city, county, and state governments that have undertaken to provide that care; the failure to provide adequate medical treatment for service veterans rests on the Federal Government and the absurd inefficiencies of its Veterans Administration hospitals (see Chapter 14); the failure to provide adequate medical care to the American Indian rests on the Federal Government's Public Health Service, which has been responsible for Indian care for more than a century.

Government's dismal record in providing health care offers a clear example of the quality of medical care that awaits all Americans if Congress adopts a program of national health insurance. All of these medical flops—the failures in providing care for the poor, the veterans and the Indians, as well as the failures of the Medicare and Medicaid programs (see Chapter 14)—are the result of precisely the sort of systems the planners would adopt for the entire nation.

The systems that failed in the above cases were presumably ideal from the vantage point of a Federal planner: care was highly centralized; fee-for-service was eliminated; patients were assigned to doctors not of their choosing; multiple specialties were housed in single facilities; treatment was rigidly controlled; physicians were salaried (critics contend that fee-for-service causes physicians to run more tests and make more patient visits than are necessary). In short, these systems were all that those who decry the "non-system" could have wanted. Each and every one of them has been a miserable failure. The system has proven costly and inefficient, and even the planners complain of the quality of care dispensed by the programs.

What is amazing is the fact that the planners are surprised by such results. Inefficiency is the nature of the system the planners envision.

Former Ohio Governor James A. Rhodes recently wrote that, "Hundreds of millions of taxpayers' dollars are being wasted every year because of cumbersome and unnecessary paperwork forced upon state and local governments by overorganized federal agencies." Rhodes based his charge on a report by the Council for Reorganization of Ohio State Government. The Council, Rhodes said, "uncovered a vast understructure of red tape, duplication and triplication that staggers the imagination."

The Council studied only six state departments, but found that those six were required to submit to the Federal Government nearly 100,000 copies of 664 separate forms each year, requiring 539,000 man-hours (the equivalent of the full time of nearly 260 state employees), at an annual cost to Ohio taxpayers of more than $2.5 million. Four departments of the city of Cincinnati alone were required to file nearly 3,000 copies of 122 forms, requiring 60,400 man-hours (the equivalent of the full time of approximately 30 city employees) at a total cost of well over a quarter of a million dollars.

"In Ohio," Rhodes said, "it is estimated that 50 percent of the

time spent on the job by welfare department employees is used to
fill out Federal forms."

A subcommittee of the U.S. House of Representatives has reported that the Federal Government now requires that citizens fill
out some 360,000 forms and questionnaires, with a quarter of a
million Federal employees chiefly involved with filing the paper
into 25 million cubic feet of filing space. According to syndicated
columnist Henry J. Taylor, "That's more than 12 times the entire
rentable floor space in the vast 102-story Empire State Building—
only for the jungle's filing cabinets."

Such is the nature of a government system.

Writing in the September, 1970, issue of *Playboy*, author Gene
Marine described the small band of men known as *cientificos* who
surrounded Mexican dictator Porfirio Diaz at the turn of this century. According to Marine, the *cientificos* saw themselves as "expert
technicians, applying 'scientific' methods to the administration of
government." Wrote Marine, "The *cientifico* mentality can't tolerate anybody who gets in the way of a simple solution to a simple
problem."

So it is with the planners who today call for a new order in
medicine—a throwing over of the free enterprise system and its
replacement with national health insurance. Though the system
they propose is complex, it stems from a ridiculously simplistic,
shoot-from-the-hip approach to problem solving. Are medical costs
too high? Disregarding inflation, increasing wages, and technological advances, today's *cientificos* propose a simple solution: replace
the non-system with a rigidly controlled, complex system.

Are there too few doctors in the run-down sections of the major
cities? Disregarding the shabby surroundings and the high crime
rates, the *cientificos* propose a simple solution: replace the "non-
system" with a system.

Fortunately, the *cientificos* don't yet have the upper hand.

"It does not appear that the American public is ready to or nearly
ready to abolish the existing system of medical care," writes Eli
Ginzberg of Columbia University, in his book *Men, Money and
Medicine*. "... one must guard against overoptimism from structural
changes," Ginzberg warns. "Medical care is expensive and will
remain expensive. The only real control over costs is to keep the
amount of medical services within bounds; to be sure that essential

needs are met but that medical services do not expand beyond."

As pointed out earlier, not only will a new government-controlled medical system *not* reduce medical costs, there is good reason to believe it will increase costs.

But there are other problems even more important. A patient wants more from a physician than salves and injections of penicillin. He wants reassurance and support. He goes needing comfort as well as medication. He needs the doctor's time and the doctor's attention. He needs the doctor's concern about him, not as a "patient" or a "disease," but as a person. That is the magic ingredient of medicine. It may not cure—but then again it may.

Elsewhere in this book I have pointed out that *almost all* American mothers give birth in a hospital, attended by a physician. In many other nations, with medical "systems," births are attended by midwives. Dr. Frank Furstenberg, a founder member of the Reuther-Kennedy Committee for National Health Insurance, participating in an American Enterprise Institute debate in Washington, D.C., complained recently that American physicians are inefficient and wasteful of their time; for example, he pointed out, if deliveries were handled by midwives, doctors would be free to spend their time on more important matters (see Chapter 1).

Perhaps. But I doubt that American women are ready to revert to the primitive days of having their babies delivered by midwives just to satisfy Dr. Furstenberg's concept of the ideal "system."

In Dr. Roth's words: "Americans, with some militance, proclaim their right to personalized, high quality, competent care." Those precious ingredients of the free enterprise "non-system" are too valuable to be given up in blind obeisance before the altar of centralized planning.

8. Doctor Scrooge

Physicians have developed a "grab-bag attitude," Louisiana Senator Russell Long cried recently. Long's accusation was part of a massive campaign to create sympathy for government health programs by undermining public confidence in the private enterprise physician.

"The image of the selfless doctor has been gradually changing, in the American mind, to that of a callous, overpaid, high-living, Cadillac-riding businessman," Daniel Schorr whines. "Dr. Kildare has dissolved into Dr. Scrooge. . . ."

Schorr was resorting to a gambit long favored by promoters of liberal schemes—couching their own criticisms in terms of *universal* complaint. The truth is, nationwide surveys have revealed a high degree of patient satisfaction with their doctors, and few complaints about the fees those doctors charge. By telling John Doe, falsely, that his neighbors are upset over the high cost of physician care, promoters of national health insurance hope to convince him that he, alone, has been receiving satisfactory care at reasonable rates, and that something must be done for the sake of his presumably discontented neighbors.

So it is with criticisms that physicians have become corrupt and greedy, gouging their patients (or, through Medicare and Medicaid, the taxpayers) for huge unearned sums of money.

Time magazine, in its issue for February 21, 1969, complained that: "The tightly organized medical profession fends off any and all attacks from the outside, and in case of complaints against any of its members, sits as prosecutor, judge and jury. It is the rare patient who even tries to protest *an obviously excessive doctor's bill*" (emphasis added).

Time's assertions do not agree with *Time's* statistics. According to the article, 150 complaints of "fee gouging" are lodged in an average year against the 7,200 members of the New York Medical Society: 150 complaints out of something like 12 million medical treatments a year (an average of 30 patients a day, five days a week, 11 months a year). By implication, *Time* asserts that (a) nearly 12 million patients are too ignorant or too insensitive to the charges they pay, to realize that they've been overcharged, or (b) 12 million patients are too intimidated by 7,200 doctors to protect themselves.

There is, of course, an alternative explanation: that most patients are satisfied with the fairness of the fees they pay for the service they receive.

Claims that private physicians are excessively greedy and commonly dishonest are frequently based on reports that a number of doctors have received substantial yearly incomes through Medicare and Medicaid fee payments, and that an IRS investigation has discovered fraud in half the physician tax returns checked. "The Watchdog staff of the Senate Finance Committee made an exhaustive study that found several thousand doctors earning more than $25,000 . . . by assembly-line treatment of Medicaid patients," Schorr wrote in his book, *Don't Get Sick in America*.

Dr. Gerald Dorman, former President of the American Medical Association, insists that the payments were earned. "There were many times when we used to care for our older patients at a lower fee, or free," he said. "The government said that there shall be no more free medicine. Everybody must be paid for it. And we have doctors, not only under Medicare, but also in Medicaid, who have made a large income because they are working with the people who are poor, who come under these programs of government care. . . .

"Now in the old days before Medicare and Medicaid," Dr. Dorman said, "these people would have been treated free or for a minimal fee. We've had people up in Harlem who were treated for a fifty-cent office fee . . . but these things have changed."

As a result of Medicare and Medicaid, physicians now collect fees for service they once performed free. It is ludicrous for the supporters of those programs to complain about the payment of those fees. Physicians, themselves, for years prior to the 1965 passage of Medicare, had warned of the inevitable consequences.

Advocates of government medical controls have made much of news media reports that physicians are gouging the public to the tune of many thousands of dollars a year. One case that has been frequently cited is that of Dr. Paul F. Maddox, a physician in Campton, Kentucky, who received $81,726 from Medicare in 1968, and more than $106,000 in 1969.

Dr. Maddox serves one of the nation's most financially depressed areas, with well over half the local families below the government's official "poverty" level. The doctor serves his community more than 12 hours a day, every day of the year, including Sundays and holidays (for example, on Thanksgiving Day, 1969, he saw 117 patients). Because there is no other doctor in the community, and no hospital within 45 miles, Dr. Maddox is on call 24 hours a day. In 1969, the year he collected $106,000 from Medicare, he cared for 49,209 patients—an average of more than 135 a day—and delivered nearly 400 babies.

To help him perform this exhausting service, Dr. Maddox employed, with his own funds, 13 full-time nursing assistants and 11 part-time physician assistants (residents at a university hospital). His overhead costs for drugs, supplies, etc., were in excess of $123,000 in 1968, the year he billed Medicare for $81,000. The next year, when he billed Medicare for $106,000, his overhead costs were approximately $150,000!

Dr. Maddox delivers babies in his clinic, and charges $70 for the delivery and eight hours in a clinic bed—at least $230 less than the cost of delivery in the distant university hospital. At that rate, Dr. Maddox saves the state $92,000 a year—more than he received from the government in 1968 and almost as much as he received in 1969.

Although Dr. Maddox does collect from Medicare and Medicaid, many of his patients are eligible for neither program, although they too have financial difficulties. In one case, he delivered five babies to a local woman and charged her $25—$5 for each delivery.

According to *American Medical News,* Dr. Maddox now has more than $200,000 in unpaid bills on his books. "I hope to collect after the Resurrection," he says simply.

Dr. Maddox is not a typical case, of course, but it is not at all uncommon for a physician to work 60 to 70 hours a week—meaning he sees more patients and thus has a higher income. For example, as mentioned earlier, a survey of the 3,200 members of the Medical Society of the County of Kings (Brooklyn), revealed that the members averaged 6.5 days of work a week, including 187 hours a year in hospital clinics treating indigent patients. In all, the county's doctors dispensed $22 million a year in free care and free medicine. That was *before* Medicare. Today, they get paid for much of that care. As a result, their incomes are higher, and the burden on the taxpayers is greater.

Critics of free enterprise medicine made Dr. Maddox, and others like him, the targets of harsh public censure. In truth, he earned every dime he was paid—and considerably more that he wasn't paid.

The facts were equally distorted in widespread news reports that the Internal Revenue Service had found frequent instances of tax fraud by physicians who received Medicare payments. According to Robert Myers, who was chief actuary of the Social Security Administration at the time, this is what actually happened:

The Social Security Administration compiled a list of medical service *providers* who had received $25,000 or more in Medicare payments. The list totaled only 11,000, including doctors, dentists, clinics and commercial suppliers of medical equipment. Only 3,000 of the 11,000 returns required IRS auditing. Of these 3,000, only 1,500 showed as much as a $100 discrepancy, the basis for further investigation. Thus, "half" the returns (1,500 out of the 3,000 audited) were reported as "fraudulent." The truth is: 1,500 of the returns checked contained *either possible fraud or possible error*—1,500 out of almost 328,000 physicians and untold numbers of dentists, clinics and medical appliance suppliers.

In fact, out of the 338,000 physicians in the United States, only *five* have been convicted of fraud in the history of Medicare, and only *five* more are now under fraud indictment. Even if all five doctors currently under indictment are found guilty, the number of dishonest physicians comes to only 10 in the entire United States, or approximately one in 33,000.

At the end of 1969, Robert M. Ball, Commissioner of the Social Security Administration, confirmed the low instance of physician cheating. "It is clear from our investigations," he said, "that the number of attempts at fraud or abuse is relatively very small." Ball went on to say that SSA investigations frequently revealed that tax discrepancies were based on clerical errors, misunderstandings or honest mistakes.

In 1971, the Internal Revenue Service reported that a study of 1968 tax returns filed by 8,400 health care providers confirmed that 99 percent of Medicare and Medicaid receipts had been accurately reported. Yet the campaign continues, based primarily in the Senate Finance Committee, the powerful legislative base for a number of leading advocates of expanded government regulation.

In September, 1970—months after Myers and Ball had revealed the truth about the "fraud" reports—the committee called Meade Whitaker, a Treasury Department employee, who repeated the disproved claim that half of the 3,000 doctors who received more than $25,000 each from the government had failed to pay taxes on a substantial part of those earnings. Using Whitaker's testimony as a wedge, the committee endorsed a plan to require insurers to list on all claims the names and Social Security numbers of all doctors receiving more than $600 a year for treating patients under the Medicare and Medicaid programs. The move would single out physicians for "suspect" status, subjecting their incomes to detailed inspection and surveillance by government computers. Even more important, in terms of immediate objectives, the Senate crackdown will serve to generate support for national health programs "as a protection against unscrupulous doctors."

Like other aspects of the make-believe medical "crisis," the attack on Dr. Scrooge is intentional, malicious and deceiving. America's doctors deserve better.

PART THREE

THE EXPERIENCE

9. On the Brink of Medical Disaster

A cartoon appeared in a British newspaper soon after Prime Minister Harold Wilson's government was defeated in 1970, showing Wilson collapsed at his desk in apparent dismay over the election results. Behind him stood an aide, speaking into a telephone. "The PM's fainted," says the aide—"get his private doctor!"

Therein lies a great irony.

Wilson, turned out of office by the British people in the midst of a national economic crisis, was the Laborite guardian of the National Health Service, the government medical program that has, in a little over 20 years, reduced the quality of British medical care to a standard so dismal that even the men who run the system prefer to get their medical care elsewhere. While the Labor government was in power the British press delighted in hurling sarcastic barbs at Wilson for using a private doctor rather than trust his care to the National Health Service for which his government takes so much credit.

Richard Crossman, Wilson's Minister of Social Services, championed the NHS and openly campaigned to wipe out Britain's few remaining vestiges of private medical practice. Writing in a pamphlet issued by the Socialist Fabian Society, Crossman publicly called the growth of private insurance in England "a disturbing element." All the while, British reports revealed, Crossman himself was a member of a private plan—and had been for a number of years.

(To be a member of a private insurance plan in England means paying double for health care: once for private insurance premiums and once for the compulsory government tax to support the National Health System. Yet two million Britons are now doing just that—paying double so they can buy care from the country's remaining private practitioners and use private hospital facilities rather than receive the poor quality of care available under the government system.)

Britain's national health system was the Labor government's political "baby"—the Socialist goal of "free" government medicine for everybody. In 23 years it had become such a costly and unmanageable failure—and had provided such poor health care—that the men who defended it on the stump had abandoned it in providing for their own medical needs. Now the British have turned the Laborites out. Prime Minister Edward Heath's Conservative government is moving, with wide support, to roll back the Socialist programs of the 1960s. The English have decided that to go forward the nation must first go backward—back from the "progressive" programs of government regulation to the almost abandoned precepts of private enterprise. The National Health Service is one of the prime candidates for early change.

Ironically, all of this is happening at the same time that American liberals are calling for a national health program in this country to emulate the pattern of the British and other Europeans.

In 1948, the year Britain instituted its National Health Service, the highly regarded Brookings Institution issued a report by George W. Bachman and Lewis Merriam that concluded: "It is apparent that the United States, under its voluntary system of medical care, has made greater progress . . . than any other country. . . . There is every reason to believe that these trends will continue unabated . . ."

The report was prophetic. The *Philadelphia Inquirer*, in a 1970 study of European medicine, reported that American doctors are much more active in preventive medicine; that the average length of confinement in American hospitals is many days shorter than in Sweden, Germany or England, all of which have national health programs; that American doctors, on the average, spend more time with each patient than do their European counterparts.

But even these conclusions fail to tell the whole story.

Government health programs throughout Europe are plagued by severe overcrowding, inadequate and often antiquated facilities, dangerously outmoded equipment, drastic shortages of personnel, lack of essential services, impersonal attention, lack of privacy and long waiting lines for admission to government hospitals. National health systems have caused a disastrous upheaval in the medical care received by hundreds of millions of Europeans.

Due to England's severe shortage of medical personnel, for example, there are no nurses in the ante-natal ward of Hemmel Hempstead Hospital after 8 P.M. Consequently, when Ellen Foster's labor pains began, after 8, she had to climb 3 flights of stone stairs, unaccompanied, to reach the labor ward. Within 18 hours after delivery she was discharged; the hospital was overcrowded and needed the bed space. To most American women, treatment such as that received by Ellen Foster would be frustrating and embittering. Despite the cries of medicine's critics in this country, Americans have come to expect far better care than that received in Britain's government hospitals. But Mrs. Foster's experience is not at all unique. Health care facilities in most European countries are far below the standards in the United States.

Dr. Joselen Ransome, a London-based hospital consultant, has become so concerned about the frustrating conditions under which the British medical profession is forced to work that he has publicly complained that the National Health System is "totally inadequate to meet the demands of ever more sophisticated medicine and surgery." Ransome's complaints included:

"1.   Out of date, often dirty buildings. In some cases there is not even a lift by which the elderly, or those with heart diseases, can reach the appropriate hospital department.

"2.   Totally inadequate building programme.

"3.   Totally inadequate programme for up-dating equipment to keep abreast of modern medical developments.

"4.   A totally inadequate programme for streamlining office procedures . . .

"5.   Totally inadequate funds for salaries, which in turn leads to:

(a) Progressive reduction in the number of nurses and thus a fall in morale of the overworked remainder.

(b) Difficulties in recruiting all grades of administrative and auxiliary staff of the right calibre, in competition with commerce and industry."

These difficulties, Ransome charged, result "in an increasing muddle and thus cumulative decline of all hospital personnel."

The facts support Dr. Ransome's frustrated observations. A recent British government report on mental hospitals in that country revealed that 40 percent are more than 100 years old, and most of the remainder are more than 80 years old—typical of the British hospital situation in general. A memorandum prepared for the Department of Health reported that some NHS patients are receiving treatment in facilities built 150 years ago—at the beginning of the 1800's. The average patient, the report said, is in a hospital that is 70 years old; only one-fourth of Britain's 2,300 hospitals were designed in the last 60 years! Anthony Lejeune, writing in the pamphlet "Socialized Medicine: Showcase of Failure," called Britain's hospitals the "oldest in the Western world." Staff accommodations are so poor, complained the board chairman of a hundred-year-old Scottish hospital, that they "would not be allowed in industry, commerce or any other sphere of public life."

Former Minister of Health Enoch Powell has stated that establishment of England's government health program had the effect of delaying and preventing a vast amount of the hospital building that would otherwise have taken place in the years immediately after World War II. Trusts and voluntary groups were eager to start building, he said, but bureaucrats and politicians had assumed the role of assigning priorities and hospitals were superseded by other building projects. As a result, between 1948, the year the National Health Service was inaugurated, and 1962, there were no new hospitals built in England. Only three were built between 1962 and 1970. And this in a nation of 55 million people!

The outmoded buildings pose hidden dangers for unsuspecting patients:

—Drainage facilities at the Victoria Hospital in Worksop are so inadequate that heavy rains early in 1970 caused crude sewage to overflow and pour through the casualty department, causing a major health hazard.

—A 19-year-old patient at Newmarket General Hospital lost an eye recently as the result of infection caused by erection of a make-shift "operating room"—a plastic tent set up on temporary rubber flooring in a recreation hall. The damp floor, inadequate and contaminated ventilation, a faulty air-gauge and sterilizer and unsterile wash basin caused infections that also struck three other patients with less permanent effects.

—A fire that killed 24 patients at Sheldon Hospital in Shrewsbury was blamed on unsafe facilities, but the Regional Hospital Board, dependent on government allocations, reported that it lacked the necessary funds to make improvements that would remove the danger.

—Sanitation restrictions are so lax at St. Stephens Hospital in Chelsea that some of the hospital's departments had to be closed after cats moved into the hospital, causing an invasion of fleas in beds, clothing, linen cupboards, consulting rooms and examination rooms.

A panel of distinguished British physicians and surgeons recently issued an urgently worded plea to the government to do something about the country's inadequate emergency services. The committee had undertaken a pilot survey on emergency care as a preliminary to a more intensive national study, but the doctors were so troubled by what they found that they decided a call for action was "a more immediate task than further surveys." Only 30 percent of Britain's hospitals have adequate emergency facilities, the committee reported, and warned that a severe shortage of doctors, nurses and other staff was forcing the closing of increasing numbers of casualty departments. According to the report, all the hospitals investigated had inadequate and outdated emergency room facilities, which were impossible to keep sterile.

Emergency hospital services have virtually collapsed around Milford Haven, a heavily industrialized area of south Wales in which there had been two major accidents in the preceding four months. Seriously injured residents of that area now have to travel up to 40 miles to reach a "district emergency center." The nearest regular hospital emergency facility is open only a few hours a day, on a makeshift basis. Doctors claim at least one patient has died because it took him so long to reach a hospital.

The situation is desperate, warned Dr. George Middleton, speaking for some 60 physicians in the area. "In the event of a major disaster at any one of the four oil refineries around Milford Haven, there is no way in which we could cope." With only seven ambulances available, the doctors estimate it would take up to four hours to get patients to Glanwili Hospital, which is to be used as the main casualty center.

The inadequacy of hospital facilities was dramatically illustrated in 1969 when David Evans, a consultant surgeon at Kent, refused to carry out a scheduled operation. "I cannot work without sufficient instruments," he told the press. "I cannot take the risk with patients' lives." Dr. Evans complained that a week earlier a thyroid operation had been held up for an hour while the operating staff tried to find a suitable syringe. "There were only three available," he said. "The first broke, the second did not work and we had to wait for the third to be sterilized."

The Secretary of the Hospital Management Committee admitted that Evans was not alone in his campaign for more and better equipment. "Most doctors are always complaining of lack of equipment—and rightly so," he said, "but only so much money is allocated . . ."

Bureaucratically determined priorities were sharply criticized following a visit to two Pembrokeshire hospitals by Ifor Davies, Under Secretary for Wales. New 20-foot flagpoles were erected at the hospitals four days before the official visit. Irate members of Parliament demanded to know who ordered the poles and how much they had cost. Meanwhile, the touring official was shown rotting woodwork, a leaky roof (he had to step over a pan put on the floor to catch rain water), and an unused lavatory that had been converted into a makeshift storage facility for pathological specimens.

Britain's government health program has resulted in such deteriorated conditions in the nation's hospitals that frustrated nurses invaded Parliament in early 1969. While the other nurses fought with male ushers trying to remove her from the gallery, Sister Patricia Veal jumped to her feet in the midst of a debate on measures to improve conditions for horses and shouted: "Nurses want to fight for the patients of this country." Other spectators applauded and cheered. Ushers finally had to drag the bitter nurses from the chambers.

"We are determined to use suffragette tactics because nobody listens to the quiet, dignified, ladylike approach any more," Sister Patricia said. "We intend to make the government realize that conditions in hospitals are deteriorating alarmingly."

Mrs. Pamela Harper knew what Sister Patricia was talking about. Her two children were born in the maternity unit at Bishops Stortfort Hospital. In a 2,000-word letter to the Hertfordshire and Essex Hospital Board, Mrs. Harper complained:

—the hospital is so old-fashioned that the many babies are born on an old couch;

—the hospital still uses old painted wooden commodes;

—there were only three toilets to serve 30 patients in the maternity ward;

—wards are cold and gloomy; patients in labor and giving birth can be heard by other expectant mothers.

The poor quality of hospital food also leads to many complaints. Crispin Gray, a senior research assistant at Cambridge, complained to authorities at Old Addenbrooke Hospital about the "awful food" served to his wife while she was a patient there. When his wife criticized the food, Gray said, a Sister agreed the meals were bad and said "If you want to get better, you ought to have some decent food brought in." As a result, Gray carried a plastic bag of food to his wife at each visiting period. In spite of the fact that his wife was four months pregnant, Gray said, she could not get any milk except with her tea.

But the outmoded facilities, inadequate equipment and sometimes frustrating treatment are not the most severe drawbacks that have resulted from government medicine. Hospitals in England and other nations with national health programs are overcrowded to an extent unknown in the United States. When Social Services Minister Richard Crossman visited Central Mental Hospital in Warwickshire, he inspected wards so full that patients had to climb over each other's beds. His report stated simply: "This hospital is overcrowded to a hopeless extent—but it's no worse than many other hospitals I have been to."

While touring a hospital near Birmingham, Mr. Crossman came to a similar situation—a ward crammed with 72 beds, twice the number it was built to accommodate. Beds in the ward were so close that their sides touched. Patients got into and out of their beds either by climbing over the foot of the bed or over the patients in adjoining beds. None of the patients had space for either a wardrobe or foot locker. Shoes had to be kept on the window sills. Night clothes were kept on the floor, stuffed under the beds. There were no flowers because there was no room for a vase. The 72 patients shared eight washbasins and three old chipped toilets.

"This is the worst overcrowding I have ever seen," Crossman said. "How can the staff do their job in conditions like these?"

Joan Hobson, writing in *Private Practice*, reported that "Emergency wards in many hospitals are overcrowded to the point where patients' beds have to be arranged along the corridors."

Melchior Palyi, in his article "How Sick is State Medicine?", chided, "Before nationalization . . . no one ever heard of a hospital advising expectant mothers (as has happened since) to apply for a bed 12 months ahead. The overload creates a need for more space and equipment, which increases the financial worries of the institutions and seriously impairs the medical and human value of the whole setup."

In a 1970 speech, Victor Goodhew, a member of the British Parliament, lashed out angrily at the low quality of his country's hospitals. "Building has been notorious in its absence in the past two decades," Goodhew said. "The meagre sums of State money which have been available have been used mainly to patch up and adapt, often most unsatisfactorily, existing old hospital buildings. The rectification of this situation somehow steadily recedes like a mirage. The effect on staff morale can be serious. Accommodation is often poor and bad working conditions may discourage, perhaps permanently, the recruitment of doctors and nurses."

The overcrowding has serious effects on the patients in hospitals, but its effect is most deeply felt by those patients who can't get in at all. Government figures in August, 1966, revealed that more than 100,000 elderly and chronically sick Britons were on the waiting lists for hospital beds. In addition, there were 76,000 women waiting to get into hospitals for gynecological treatment; 80,000 children waiting to have their tonsils removed; 30,000 patients awaiting ophthalmic surgery; 22,000 awaiting plastic surgery. By the end of 1968 there were more than half a million British patients awaiting admission to hospitals, 71 percent of them in need of surgery.

Dr. Edward L. McNeil, a British-trained physician and surgeon who now practices in Mt. Kisco, New York, has described why he left England:

". . . My first 'house job' was as House Surgeon in a London hospital . . . There was rarely an empty bed and I had the unpleasant task of turning down at least two out of three requests by GP's for emergency admissions . . .

"I later learned what it was like to be a GP trying to have a patient admitted for an emergency condition, telephoning five or six different hospitals without success, then, in frustration, sending the patient to the emergency department of a hospital that had already turned down a request for admission, and hoping for the best."

In later years, McNeil wrote, London instituted an Emergency Bed Service "to which a GP could direct his requests for admission and they would call all the hospitals for him, then force the hospital they considered most able to adapt to an extra admission to take the patient."

"This system was fine in theory," McNeil said, "but in practice it would often take the EBS six to twelve hours to find a bed, and some patients could not wait that long."

McNeil had already experienced the space shortage; as a young house surgeon he had run into frustrated GP's who had done the same thing he was to do later—sending patients to an emergency room after receiving an official turndown. "Such bad manners," he had thought at the time—"I had already told him on the telephone that I didn't have any empty beds and we had seven extra beds up in the corridors and down the middle of the ward!"

There is a waiting list for many operations, McNeil writes. "One to two years is not uncommon." One patient in the Birmingham area applied for an operation in 1962 and was finally admitted to a hospital seven years later.

To supplement his meager income as a general practitioner, McNeil began to "moonlight," accepting a job as clinical assistant in the Royal National Throat, Nose and Ear Hospital in London. "One of my duties was to help re-evaluate those children on the waiting list to have their tonsils removed, to see if they should be moved up the list or onto the list with less priority. Some had been on the list six years. At the time I left, the theoretical waiting time was ten years."

The shortage of hospital space is a natural result of the inevitable massive demand for "free" medical care. Within less than three years after Britain's national health program went into effect, the Ministry of Health had announced (on December 1, 1950) that 553,557 people were on the waiting list for hospital beds—100,-000 of them in London alone. The problem leads to frightening results. As a group of health administrators informed the (London) Institute of Public Administration shortly after the NHS went into effect, "The public is adopting the attitude that because of the Welfare State they have no responsibilities for their aged parents." As a result, they reported, many of the mentally deficient and the helpless aged were left without care and had to shift for themselves, since there was no room in the overcrowded hospitals.

On April 18, 1951, in a speech in the House of Lords, Lord Saltoun reported 17 known cases "of old people who were found dead in varying conditions of horror." As Melchior Palyi described the situation, "The problem of the overcrowded hospitals is to keep out the old and chronically ill whom they cannot discharge."

"Hurry up and wait" is an old gag. The British have adopted half of it, and it's not funny. "Wait" seems to be the watchword of government medicine.

An independent association designed to protect patients' rights is pressing the government to investigate a hundred cases of people who have been waiting for hospital treatment for over a year, some of them for several years. The association itself is looking into at least 200 similar cases.

"Need a childless woman within sight of the end of her safe child-bearing years apologize for seeking to shorten the wait for a small operation that might overcome her infertility?" the association asked. "Should a mother of eight children have to wait 18 months for sterilization?" The association complained that many patients were told they could have the operations they need, immediately, as paying private patients; they are understandably upset, having paid compulsory government health taxes for many years.

When the offers do come, they often border on the absurd: one man received a telegram at 5:30 P.M. one day in July, 1969, notifying him that a bed was available for him at 10 the next morning—in a hospital 200 miles from his home. To take the bed, he would

PART THREE: THE EXPERIENCE

have had to find someone else to take his work, and arrange for transportation—an impossible task on so short notice. Consequently the bed went to someone else and at last report, a year and a half later, he was still waiting for his operation.

Harold Gurden, a member of Parliament from Birmingham, has called for a public investigation into waiting lists for children to have ear operations. In 1969, Gurden said, 50 Birmingham children a year were going permanently deaf because they were unable to receive hospital treatment in time. The situation has not improved.

David Rhydderch, chairman of the Birmingham Health Council, called the problem a "national scandal." "Hospitals throughout Britain have nearly 80,000 children on their waiting lists for treatment," he said.

"Children face total deafness because of the waiting list," a consultant at a Birmingham hospital told reporters recently. "It is a very sad situation."

For Americans, accustomed to fairly rapid hospital admission, the half-million people waiting to get into British hospitals may be the best indicator of all as to what changes may be expected if government health programs are adopted here.

Hospitals, however, are not the only victims of government medicine. Medical facilities throughout Britain have declined at a disastrous rate. The handicap under which deaf children must labor, for example, has been increased by a severe shortage of new hearing aids in Britain, largely the result of increased demand for "free" health appliances. Joan Hobson has reported that at the end of 1970 one Birmingham school for the deaf was awaiting a long overdue supply of 140 hearing aids. At another school, the headmaster complained: "We have got to the stage where there is just not a supply of aids, and this sometimes lasts for months. I had a letter from the Ministry (months ago) saying that problems with supply had been overcome and we had no cause to worry, but we are still waiting. We wonder just how long this can go on. The effect on the children's education could be absolutely disastrous in later life. The early period of teaching for deaf children is considered to be the most vital if they are to overcome their handicap."

Britain's national health program has resulted in a serious deterioration of facilities in doctors' offices, too. As a means of cutting costs, bureaucrats in some British health offices have ordered doctors to share their office space with other people. For example, four doctors operating a Health Centre near London have complained that a welfare clinic, a chiropody service for the aged, and blood donor sessions take over their offices in the afternoons. A Health Centre designed for Lanarkshire is to be provided, with the government stipulation that whenever any doctor is not in his offices they will be used by someone else.

Sometimes the office-sharing results in complications; for example, a Flintshire doctor recently arrived at the building he and five colleagues share, reluctantly, with an ante-natal clinic, to find his door locked and a sign stating that the offices had been closed "owing to infectious disease in the clinic." The six doctors had to find new office space in nearby private houses and leave tracing instructions for their patients.

Dr. McNeil recalls the office facilities with which he had to treat his patients while practicing in England.

"Not having any X-ray facilities in the office, and less than meagre lab equipment, and little or no time for workup tests, any patient seen who needed these tests had to be referred to the hospital clinics. A very few simple tests could be referred directly to the hospital lab (mainly those concerned with the diagnosis and treatment of TB) but anything approaching a blood chemistry, an EKG or an X-ray could not be ordered by the GP directly, so the patient had to be referred to the appropriate clinic for those doctors running the clinic to decide on the tests and order them.

"The result of this angle of the system, plus the difficulty of obtaining a hospital bed for acute conditions such as myocardial infarction, pneumonia and stroke (especially stroke), meant that a GP treated many of these conditions in the patient's home without any of the ancillary diagnostic aids which would be routine in a hospital. I recognized the satisfaction of 'curing' a condition with minimal help of diagnostic equipment and lab tests, but there was always that sneaking suspicion at the back of my mind that the patient may not have had the condition I thought I had cured.

"Without this confirming knowledge, there was no testing of one's diagnostic and therapeutic ability and so improving one's effectiveness as a physician.

"With my present knowledge of cardiac arrhythmias which can

be prevented or ameliorated by information only to be gained from ancillary equipment, I shudder at the risks the patients ran under my care."

When he came to the United States to practice, McNeil writes, "My office was equipped in a manner that would have been only a dream in England. The advantages of having a lab, X-ray equipment, physiotherapy equipment, an EKG machine and an examining table that was designed to allow proper posturing of the patient were great luxuries to me. They allowed me to offer services to my patients that, to obtain under NHS, they would have had to shuffle from clinic to clinic and hospital to hospital, hardly ever knowing who the doctor was who examined them."

Much of the inadequacy of the health facilities available to the British public can be traced to the inefficiencies and incompetence of the professional bureaucracies that dominate any government program. At the end of 1969 and beginning of 1970, an epidemic of Hong Kong flu spread throughout England, taking 7,000 lives in four weeks. Angry British doctors charged that government bureaucrats in the Ministry of Health contributed to the awesome death count. "We were led to believe that any flu would not be too bad; it took us by surprise," cried Dr. R.H.M. Baines, head of the Midland Health Committee. "We were not warned in time."

Dr. Baines charged that although an available vaccine gave about 70 percent protection, the Ministry generally refused to pay for doctors to give their patients the innoculations. Since British doctors are not permitted to charge NHS patients for treatment, they would have had to buy the vaccine themselves and administer it to their thousands of patients at their own expense, an impossible undertaking in England where doctors are poorly paid state employees. Vaccine production that could have been used to save lives in England, was exported to New Zealand, South Africa and the Middle East, leaving British doctors with inadequate supplies to stem the spreading tide of death throughout the island.

An analysis of the effect of government health programs must invariably center around the British example, since advocates of national health insurance in this country frequently point to the experience of the English as a basis for their demands that the United States "get in step." But the low grade of medical facilities in England is not at all unique; experience tends to confirm that such a deterioration of medical standards follows wherever government takes over the provision or financing of health care.

The National Health Service in England is completely socialized. It is the next step beyond the national health insurance plan that has been proposed in this country as a lever to bring about the complete change of our medical care system. The French Health Service, on the other hand, does not go quite so far as the proposed American system. A social security plan, similar to a universal Medicare proposal offered by Senator Jacob Javits, of New York, the French system reimburses patients for a large part of their medical expenses, but does not offer complete coverage, as the Kennedy national health insurance plan would do, nor does it socialize much of the medical system as the British plan has done. The experience in France, then, offers a good test as to whether the failings of the NHS in providing health care facilities are a result of the greater extent to which that system has gone, or an inevitable result of any government health plan that substitutes ostensibly "free" medicine for "fee" medicine.

With government picking up much of the medical tab, French citizens are encouraged to make excessive demands on the facilities of the nation's hospitals and the time of its doctors. As in England, overutilization is a major problem.

"Most of the time I try to deal with the family illness myself," a Paris housewife told a British reporter recently. "It's far less painful than going through the red tape and administrative muddles . . ."

"Greediness for what people consider their fair share of medical care is ruining this country," complained Andre Chenue, one of the best-known art experts in Paris.

Joan Hobson describes the government-run dispensaries at which the poor are treated by state-employed doctors: "Here there is no choice of doctor and very little in the way of consultation because it is only possible to give a minimum of time to each of the hundreds of people who attend." She reported finding one of the dispensaries "in a shabby back street" of Paris. It had a decor "reminiscent of a public lavatory," she wrote. "Dejected men and women shuffled in and sat on hard benches for two or three hours to get a couple of minutes' medical attention."

Hospital accommodations are desperately short. As in Russia, with its five-year plans, and Red China, with its "great leaps forward," the French are constantly setting major national goals and laying down deadlines for accomplishing them. Under the Fifth National Plan (1966–1970) the government promised the French people that it would increase the total number of hospital beds by 100,000 (which was estimated to be one-third the number actually needed), but at the end of 1970 the plans had still not been carried out.

"French hospitals are only useful when the illness is a minor one and the period of stay brief," charged a professor at the Sorbonne. He described his own hospitalization experience in a government institution built more than 150 years ago, and very little improved since then. He swore then never again to entrust his care to government hospitals. "I am convinced that lack of privacy combined with overcrowding worsened my condition and prolonged my illness," he said. "It's better to pay for private clinic treatment and be assured of accommodation and care in line with twentieth-century progress."

Whereas most Americans can count on being hospitalized within a short distance from their homes, the French patient often has to be treated many miles away from home and family.

"Public criticism of socialized medicine is now so much a part of French life that a weekly radio hour is devoted to a listener-participation program in which dissatisfied patients air their grievances," Mrs. Hobson reported.

The French example is a clear indication that it is government medicine itself—not the particular form which is adopted—that sends the standards of medical quality plunging to levels far below those that are expected by most Americans.

Other nations also have their problems with national health programs:

Dr. T.R. Marshall, an associate professor at the University of Kentucky, visited Japan in October, 1969, and reported: "The hospitals are fairly small, poorly equipped and extremely crowded. The outpatient clinics are overflowing with patients, and the service and care are very similar to those of the National Health System in England."

At the time Dr. Marshall visited Japan, the nation's doctors were on strike against the National Health System. Less than two years later, in July, 1971, 60,000 Japanese doctors walked out again.

Sweden, too, has felt the brunt of a national health program. At the time Swedish medicine was nationalized, 70 percent of the nation's population was covered by private insurance programs— a situation strikingly similar to that in America, where an even higher number are protected by private companies. "In the name of equality," writes Allan C. Brownfeld, "those 70 percent were forced into a compulsory government-administered program in order to provide for the remaining 30 percent of the population not privately insured."

The results, Brownfeld reports, were the same as they have been in other countries that have adopted national health programs:

"Today there is hardly a single hospital in Sweden where there are not long waiting lists for all kinds of hospital care. It is estimated that in Stockholm hospitals alone there are more than 4,000 persons waiting to enter hospitals, 1,800 for operations. In some cases, waiting periods for minor operations may be more than half a year.

"The same situation exists not only for surgery, but for internal medicine, outpatient clinics, neurological sections, and various specialization clinics. The situation is worse in state-administered mental hospitals where there were 800 patients waiting for entrance in 1964, a situation which has since become even more critical. Extended care hospitals, nursing homes and homes for the aged are desperately understaffed and overcrowded. In some cases, there are waiting lists numbering 2,000 persons."

Discussing the medical situation in his native country, Nils Eric Brodin said: "Technically speaking, medical care is good in Sweden, but it is the overcrowded conditions and the shortage of doctors and nurses which has, in effect, lowered the health standards severely. Diagnosis is often hasty and inadequate, and much time is spent in paper work required by the state medical plan's bureaucracy."

As Brownfeld points out, Sweden has one of the highest standards of living in Europe, with adequate educational facilities and no scars of recent war. What, he wonders, has brought about these conditions of which Brodin and other Swedes complain?

One of the major problems, as in the other national health systems, has been the tremendous increase in use of hospital facilities. The number of hospital beds in Sweden increased by 25 percent while the population was increasing by only 10 percent—yet the facilities couldn't keep up and the shortage grew increasingly severe. Between 1960 and 1970, Sweden doubled the number of doctors in the country and tripled the number of nurses; yet they are unable to cope with the massive demand.

"The increase in the utilization of existing facilities comes from those who demand 'hospital vacations,'" Brodin explains. "When the tensions of life or home get too intense, many will 'rest up' in a hospital. Often a patient stays in a hospital a week before he is diagnosed . . .'I'm paying for it . . . I've got it coming' is the attitude."

Early in Sweden's experience with its national health program, Dr. Dag Knuttson, head of the Swedish medical association, estimated that half the patients in the country's hospitals "need not be there." Ironically, it has lately been suggested that Swedish patients be required to pay their own hospital bills to eliminate the pressure on the system.

No medical system is more completely nationalized than that of the Soviet Union. Dr. Russell Roth, who recently returned from a tour of Russia, wrote that Russian hospitals are "drab utilitarian structures, lacking in decor, and in most elements of staff or patient comfort. There are virtually no private rooms except for isolation purposes. Most of them, even though newly constructed, quickly acquire an air of obsolescence with cracking plaster, battered wooden floors, corroded plumbing and peeling paint . . .

"Outside of the (upper-bracket research) institutes, the equipment is, by American standards, outmoded and inadequate."

Life magazine has described medicine in Russia as 50 years behind the American system—a finding largely confirmed by Dr. Garland Campbell, one of a group of Kansas physicians who toured the Soviet Union in July and August of 1968. "We found the hospitals in Leningrad to be unbelievably barren," Dr. Campbell wrote. "Only one ward, in one of the hospitals we visited, was clean. The remainder had a definite odor and maintenance was under par. Laboratories were very skimpily equipped and would compare with one of our laboratories of about 30 to 40 years ago. The second hospital we visited had only been occupied for 10 years but the deterioration, as manifested by rotting wood around the doors and window sills, lack of paint and accumulation of debris

upon the pipes and in the corners, had to be seen to be believed
. . ."

From Leningrad the doctors went to Moscow, where they visited
an 1,100-bed hospital, including the operating room. "Two operations were in process in the same operating room," Campbell reported. One of the patients was receiving a blood transfusion
through a length of rubber tubing. "We inspected the rubber tubing later," Campbell said, "and found it to be old and friable. It had
obviously been sterilized many times." (In the United States rubber
tubing became obsolete about 1940 because it could not be adequately cleaned and re-sterilized and the percentage of reaction
from its use was unacceptably high.)

"We saw rather sophisticated medical equipment in the public
museum," he said, "but did not see any in the hospitals we visited."

Later Campbell and the other doctors were shown an emergency
ward: "The beds . . . were approximately 18 inches from the floor,
the mattress was thin . . . There was no electrical connection or call
system from the patient to any central nursing desk.

"As a consequence of our three-week visit in Europe, one week
of which was spent in Russia, we were convinced that the medicine
available to the average European citizen is at least 30 to 35 years
behind that in the United States," Dr. Campbell wrote. "It seems
impossible that the quality of medicine in Europe can accelerate fast
enough to catch [up with] that in the United States, but as we
become more nationalized and restricted in our freedom of practice, we can lag behind enough that medicine in America and
Europe may one day be equal."

Germany has had long experience with government medicine—
dating back to Europe's first national health program, instituted by
Bismarck in the early 1880's. Dr. Klaus Rentzsch, a Hamburg
specialist, describes the results:

"Although Germany has more hospital beds per number of inhabitants than the U.S., all hospitals are overcrowded throughout
the year . . . A system of social security and medical care becomes
like a snowball as soon as it is installed; the demands rise steadily;
the snowball keeps rolling and becomes bigger and bigger; finally,
nobody can stop it." (The medical situation in Germany is discussed
more fully in the next chapter.)

One of the most severe drawbacks to good medical care under national health programs stems from the inevitable shortage of doctors, nurses and other trained personnel—a shortage caused by two prime factors:

(a) even if the number of health professionals remains constant, or is artificially increased as has been the case in Sweden, the supply is still unable to keep up with the rapidly growing demand;

(b) many doctors, frustrated by the poor quality of medical care and rigid governmental controls, either flee to other countries or quit the practice of medicine altogether.

During the 1930's—prior to the inauguration of the National Health Service—an average of 27 doctors a year left Britain to practice in Australia. In the last 10 years the rate has been about 225 a year. In 1960, 162 British doctors came to the United States to practice—more in that one year than in the entire decade of the 1930's.

Dr. Edward McNeil reports that for a number of years more than 500 doctors were leaving the United Kingdom each year. In 1970 another 400 left. "A few years ago, my old medical school sent a list of all the old students," he writes. "Reading down the list I counted that more than half of those that graduated in my class had left England or the practice of medicine." The reasons are varied: McNeil left largely because "It became clear to me that if I remained a GP under the NHS I would be practicing medicine at an unsatisfactory level both from the point of view of my own lack of opportunities to improve my abilities, and from the point of view of my patients, as there seemed few ways of improving the quality of medical care being given." Dr. Patrick O'Kelly, on the other hand, left in 1967 because New York's Memorial Hospital offered him $24,000 a year as a consultant in radiotherapy—10 times as much as he was earning in England.

The shortage of medical personnel is a familiar part of government health programs throughout Europe. While the U.S. has one doctor for every 640 citizens, more than any other major western nation, France has one for every 750 and Britain one for every 1,150 (about half the U.S. ratio). In Sweden, an effort to provide more doctors has cut medical studies by two years (a practice that many critics feel may result in a general lowering of the profession's standards and competence), and interns and students have been pressed into treatment of patients to meet the shortage.

The shortage necessarily has serious effects on the treatment received by patients. In Britain's mental hospitals, for example, a recent report revealed that there was only one psychiatrist available for every 693 patients, with the consequent lack of time for individual consultation and treatment. Recently the shortage became so severe that H.N. Rose, chairman of the Essex Executive Council, issued a plan to patients not to bother GP's with frivolous requests. In the English town of Skelmersdale New Town, in Lancashire, a housewife publicly offered the parlor of her home for use as a doctor's office if one would come to the town. Hundreds of the town's residents must now travel for three hours to reach medical care.

In Doncaster, the steady decrease in the number of family doctors caused a great deal of consternation among patients who found themselves bounced from list to list among the town's physicians. First, two doctors in a five-man group left England. One of the spots was filled, but the new man resigned after only two months, choosing consultant work to the rigors of English general practice. Finally a senior member of the group took over the list, but then he, too, notified the patients that he couldn't be responsible for their care, and transferred them to yet another doctor.

So many of the hospital staff positions in England have to be filled by immigrant doctors, unfamiliar with the English language, that members of Parliament have begun to talk of requiring English proficiency examinations before allowing doctors to practice in that country. A number of British hospitals now require language tests before permitting overseas doctors to take staff appointments.

"It has become obvious that there are a number of doctors working in hospitals whose knowledge of English is inadequate for the work they do," warned the Junior Doctors' Hospital Association. "Also the medical training of some foreign doctors is so different from that of UK graduates that it is impossible for them to practice competently in the relatively unsupervised posts they occupy."

More and more, however, the foreign graduates are finding positions as assistants to family doctors who are forced to overlook the possible dangers that may result from failures of communication. The fact is, there just are not enough British doctors to fill the positions. One London suburban doctor, for example, recently reported that his advertisement for an assistant received 67 replies, but only one applicant was British. Of the others, 58 were either Indian or Pakistani, five were Nigerian, and the others were Irish, Australian and Chinese.

Even this stopgap availability of medical personnel may soon be removed, however. India is faced with a massive doctor shortage of its own, and there is a mounting campaign in that nation to recall Indian doctors practicing overseas. A spokesman for the British Medical Association has warned that removal of the Indian doctors, who provide much of Britain's health manpower, would seriously endanger the National Health System.

British patients pay heavily for the toll government medicine has taken on the number of physicians practicing in that country.

In 1969, three-year-old Scott Veitch fell in the garden of his home in Gravesend. Scott's mother rushed him to a nearby hospital where he was X-rayed and doctors diagnosed a double fracture. The child then had to wait in severe pain for *seven hours* until an anesthetist arrived. In reply to a formal complaint, the Hospital Group Secretary answered: "The anesthetist was delayed at another hospital . . . It was very unfortunate but when we have only one anesthetist for a number of hospitals this sort of situation is bound to happen."

Despite the obvious need, especially in the field of general practice, fewer and fewer young doctors are willing to subject themselves to the burdens of Britain's national health program. "Urgent steps need to be taken to attract more young doctors into general practice if Britain is to avoid 'a critical shortage' in 20 or 30 years," the *Medical News Tribune* reported. But despite this prediction of an impending "crisis," a survey released in mid-1970 by the Royal College of General Practitioners revealed "a fall in the proportions of young general practitioners and an increase in the middle-aged (40–55) group."

The problem is not limited to Great Britain. Health Minister Camillo Ripamonti recently revealed that a drastic nursing shortage in Italian hospitals has forced physicians to perform nursing duties during operations.

The nursing situation in England is just as bad. Officials have begun recruiting overseas for women to take up nursing positions in British hospitals, and married and retired nurses have been

urged to return to work. The situation shows no sign of improvement. A new half-million-dollar, 200-bed wing was completed at
Corbett Hospital in Stourbridge during 1970, but the wing was
unusable because there were no nurses to staff it.

Other health services have also been hard hit. An article in London's *Medical News Tribune*, in October, 1970, reported that between 95 and 100 dentists leave England each year, "while the
influx of foreign dentists is nowhere near high enough to keep pace
with the exodus."

The article reported on a survey published in the *British Dental
Journal* that revealed that 31 percent of the emigrating dentists
head for Australia, 22 percent for Canada, 15 percent for South
Africa, 6 percent for the United States and 5 percent for New
Zealand. "At least half of these are believed to be staying abroad
permanently," the article said. "In contrast, although an average of
135 foreign dentists enter Britain every year, almost as many are
thought to be returning home. Only a small number stay in Britain
for any length of time . . ."

Hospital pharmacists in the Liverpool region recently reported
that they could no longer guarantee minimum standards of safety
unless something was done soon to relieve staff shortages in their
profession. The Guild of Public Pharmacists reported that the hospital pharmaceutical service had become largely dependent upon
young and inexperienced trainees and part-time help, and argued
that hardly any career pharmacists had been recruited into the
service during the past 10 years. Frustrated, the pharmacists threatened a mass strike unless the government authorized a 60 percent
increase in salaries and a pay raise structure that would make the
service attractive enough to lure new high-caliber recruits.

The staff shortages, poor facilities and overcrowding have had a
serious effect on the quality of care received by European patients.
The situation is sometimes comical, but often serious.

When 66-year-old William Osbourne of Richmond, Surrey, was
injured in an auto accident, he made his way on foot to a nearby
hospital, only to be turned away. The casualty department was just
not equipped to give *any* care—not even bandaging—outside its
posted hours (9 to 5 on weekdays; 9 to noon on Saturdays). After
a long wait, Osbourne, bleeding from a deep head wound, was
finally taken to another hospital for treatment.

A similar incident happened to a man who was struck by a car outside Epsom hospital after visiting a patient there. He lay bleeding and seriously injured for nearly half an hour because hospital rules prevented the staff from helping anyone outside the hospital walls. The hospital's only ambulance was already out on a call, so another vehicle had to be summoned from four miles away to carry the injured man the 20 yards into the hospital building.

When nine-year-old Stephen Miles was operated on for appendicitis recently, his parents were told they'd have to pick him up at overcrowded Redhill General Hospital the day after the operation and drive him to a children's hospital, where they were told they'd have to furnish their own blankets and find a wheelchair so they could wheel him to a ward themselves.

Such incidents are typical of the situation throughout the country. Ernest Vine, a British army major, who recently retired to a cottage in Cardiganshire, complains: "I'd never have moved to the country if I'd realized the damned inadequacy of the medical facilities there."

Economist Arthur Seldon, writing in a British medical magazine, recently laid the blame for England's deteriorating medical care squarely at the doorstep of the government health program:

"The NHS stultifies preventive medicine by its ritual dogma that access to medical care should be equal for everyone," he said. "This is a recipe for paralysis. Experimentation with preventative techniques cannot set the pace for others to follow if nothing can be done unless it can be done for all. If this had been the rule in the last century, medical science would have been stifled in its infancy. And since a medical service financed collectively by public revenue cannot politically declare the contrary principle—that some people in some surgeries (doctors' offices) or hospitals in some parts of the country may have to benefit before other people in other surgeries in other parts—it must at best slow down the rate of innovation of new techniques . . ."

The consequent decline in the rate of technical advancement has a serious effect on the citizens whose medical care is dependent upon the competence of the national health service. For example, miners in Hucknall, Nottinghamshire, recently were forced to initiate fund-raising soccer matches and brass-band concerts to gather the nearly $1,500 it took for one of their fellow miners, Jeff Crich, to bring his young son, Darren, to the United States for brain treatment. The NHS simply had no comparable treatment for brain damage.

In another case, because there was no NHS facility available to treat brain damage suffered by a young Welsh boy, authorities placed the boy in an institution for delinquents.

A major drawback to the care available under government health programs is the lack of individual treatment and the lack of concern for the patient as a person, rather than as a statistic. The Library of Congress Legislative Reference Service, using figures from Brookings Institution's report, "Doctors, Patients and Health Insurance," drew this comparison of the time doctors spend with their patients in the U.S. and in England: "Assuming . . . that each patient on the British doctor's panel of 2,300 is seen four times a year, this would amount to 9,200 visits annually. It is estimated that a typical general practitioner in the U.S. sees 25 to 30 patients a day, amounting to 6,000 to 7,000 a year."

Using these figures, and assuming that doctors in Britain and the U.S. spend approximately the same amount of time each day in patient care, the British doctor spends 25 to 35 percent less time with each patient than his American counterpart.

One doctor, P.A.T. Wood, recently complained in a speech that "state medicine has resulted in overcrowded wards, inadequate staff and insufficient time for doctors to listen and examine their patient."

The lack of individual concern can often result in a haphazard approach that may, in serious cases, prove highly dangerous or fatal. One such result occurred recently in Southall when a hospital learned that a Mrs. Barrar needed to be notified to cut down on the anti-clotting drug that had been prescribed for her. Attendants at the hospital casually sent Mrs. Barrar a note, second class; it arrived four days later, by which time she had died from the medication. "First class mail should always be used for urgent instructions," the coroner reminded.

The excessive demand for "free" care also reduces the care available to those who really need it. A young doctor in Caernarvon, North Wales, recently wrote to a local Executive Council complaining that 18 months of practicing in the area had broken his spirit. "I regret to say that, thanks to the efforts of a hardcore of 'professional patients,' a great deal of the work is completely trivial and not worth the attention of a doctor. These people hamper me in treating the genuinely sick . . . I cannot stay in a practice where I am sacrificing my own standards of work to deal with trivia.

"I had some tremendous rows with some of the patients," he said. "I pointed out that they were visiting the Surgery far too often, but my words were like water off a duck's back."

When the doctor announced his plans to move to another practice, 200 miles away, a spokesman for the Executive Council said "We have every sympathy with the doctor in connection with this very real problem . . . but it is not confined to this area."

Bureaucratic regulations under government medical systems have a dangerous limiting effect on the physician's freedom to prescribe the treatment dictated by his training and experience. When a British doctor recently ordered gluten-free bread for a dying patient, Ministry clerks decided the bread was unnecessary and required the doctor to pay for it out of his own pocket. And when a dermatologist prescribed a medicated soap for two children suffering from scabies, the government decided the treatment was not covered under NHS policy and deducted the cost from the doctor's next paycheck. Obviously British physicians will hesitate to prescribe these treatments in the future.

The decline in standards of medical care is not limited to England. Commenting on the Soviet system, *Life* magazine observed: "To achieve quantity, the quality of treatment often suffers."

Dr. Marshall, reporting on his tour of Japan, observed: "There is no doctor-patient relationship, and a patient is shuffled from doctor to doctor and clinic to clinic frequently, with no one caring what happens to him."

In Russia and in Holland, most babies are still delivered by midwives with only simple equipment—a frightening prospect for twentieth-century American women, most of whom have become accustomed to skilled medical delivery in a hospital.

In Red China, medicine has reverted to the ancient ways of the witch doctor. "To be a doctor in Red China today is to dispense snakes pickled in oil which are sold as cure-alls in the pharmacies . . . A man is labeled a doctor if he has studied pulse-taking under a Buddhist monk for 14 months . . . Herbology is rampant . . .

Internal diseases are blamed on 'The Seven Passions'; external diseases on 'The Six Excesses,' " reports *Physician's Management* magazine.

Medicine in France, too, has suffered from the impact of its national health program. One Paris doctor, Raoul Allemand, complains: "I didn't study for seven years to spend the major part of my day filling in certificates, making out receipts and explaining the ramifications of System procedure to my patients. Every consultation involves me in completion of at least four forms. Time spent in such trivia results in less attention to patients who really need medical attention."

Paris dentists, too, are forced to give reduced quality of care. "The margin of profit on dentures is so narrow," says one, "that in order not to work at a loss we must use inferior materials which quickly disintegrate."

Obviously the patient pays a high price for the "free" medical care he receives under government health programs. Professor John Jewkes, a member of a royal commission on health care, has reported: "The average American now has more medical services than the average Briton, and the gap between the two has been widening since the inception of the National Health Service."

As a result, patients have turned to other means of receiving health treatment—even if it means paying a large additional cost. When Britain nationalized medicine in 1948, the country's private health insurance companies began to wind up their operations, figuring that there would be little market for private policies since the citizen was already forced to pay a government tax for care under the compulsory national health system. Yet the British United Provident Association (BUPA), a non-profit company that is the largest of the private health insurers in Britain, doubled its membership to 86,000 in 1949, after the British people had experienced only one year of the NHS.

Today Britain's private insurance companies are enjoying an unexpected success; two million Britons are paying double to ensure that they will receive the better care which is available under private medicine (see page 136).

"Equal health care for all NHS patients soon became firmly established," Joan Hobson reports. "Patients were now 'cases' instead of individuals. They were hurried or dawdled along, according to the speed at which local convey-belts of care were operating at any given time. Available accommodation and limited staff just couldn't cope with the pressure of work. Self-employed persons who experienced time-wasting delays complained bitterly that running their own businesses on such lines would result in swift bankruptcy.

"Membership advances a patient's status to that of a VIP who can arrange treatment at a time convenient to his domestic or business commitments. In consultation with his GP, he is able to choose the specialists he prefers and be certain of that consultant's personal attention. He has freedom of choice in selecting a nursing home or private hospital ward, obtains early admission, and can opt for a private room with TV, bedside phone and flexible visiting hours.

"In contrast, only half of the NHS patients needing a specialist actually see the consultant of their choice. In many cases they are unable to find out the name of the person who eventually does perform their operation. Private rooms are virtually unobtainable to them and a patient may be ordered into a hospital far distant from his home."

As a result, though BUPA does little advertising, it is gaining members at the rate of 6,000 families a month and in late 1970 reached a membership total exceeding 1.5 million. Though membership costs between $65 and $106 a year, on top of the compulsory government tax, a good many Britons apparently feel they cannot afford to be without the private coverage.

"A good surgeon will act with the same care either way, but where private insurance makes all the difference in the world is the speed with which you are admitted," a policyholder wrote to the association after payment of a claim. "I enquired what was the difference in the main and the answer was 'Privately; 3 to 5 days, but in the NHS, months and sometimes years.' So I asked a Sister what happened to those who simply could not afford to be dealt with privately; her reply was that many go blind if the operation (as in my case) is retinia."

By 1957—after less than 10 years in competition with government medicine—BUPA had accumulated enough of a reserve to open the first of its own nursing homes. There are now 17, each with a full range of diagnostic equipment and surgical facilities. The 544 beds in BUPA's "mini hospitals" equal more than 10 percent of the private beds in the entire nation.

Although speed of admission and care is the prime drawing card for frustrated NHS patients, the lack of privacy available under the government program also leads many to join the private insurance plans. One British builder, reveling in the luxuries that most American patients take for granted, bragged recently that in the BUPA nursing home where he was being treated he had "a private suite with bathroom and toilet."

"I have my own TV set for entertainment and a phone to maintain contact with home and business," he said, drawing the parallel between the BUPA facility, which is much like most private American hospitals, and the facilities provided by government medicine. "Facilities here are 500 percent better than some of the NHS hospitals. I've visited patients in public wards that are reminiscent of Dickensian workhouses.

"In my opinion good nursing is impossible without privacy," he said, "and that's non-existent if you are surrounded by 20 or 30 other patients."

Another insurance program, the Private Patients' Plan, now has 318,000 members and is growing at a rate of 16 percent per year. Ian Preston is one of the new policyholders. He joined after an overcrowded NHS hospital shuffled his young wife (34 years old) into a geriatric ward. Though her illness was not severe, she returned home plagued by severe mental depression as a result of the several deaths that had taken place in the ward during her hospitalization.

Eric Mills, owner of an interior decorating business, summed up the reasons that have led such a large number of Britons to incur the double cost of maintaining a private health policy in addition to the forced payments into the government program: "Any man who appreciates his responsibilities to family and colleagues is an optimistic fool not to take out cover for the superior health care made possible outside the NHS," he said.

It is important to remember that the low standards of medical care that have driven two million Britons back to the protection of private health plans—at a considerable increase in personal cost—are not the result of the particular program of government medicine that was adopted in England in 1948. The basic problems that have plagued the NHS—overcrowding, long waiting lists for hos-

pital admission, inadequate facilities, doctor shortages, hurried consultations, irritating and harmful bureaucratic regulation, lack of
privacy and cut-rate medical care—have been equally present in the
national health programs of Japan, Sweden, Germany, France and
the Soviet Union. Government medical programs have been tried
in the United States, and have produced the same results (see
Chapter 14).

Experience has proven national health programs to be failures
wherever they have been tried. Completely socialized medicine has
provided dismally inadequate health care in the Soviet Union and
in England; France has had the same results with a program of
national health insurance. The fault is not in the planning, but in
the concept. Neither bureaucrats nor legislators are equipped,
either by training or experience, to make competent judgements in
the field of medicine. Tax funds cannot provide enough beds or
enough medical facilities to handle the floodtide of demands
created by "free" medical care.

If the United States adopts a national health program—whether
the national health insurance plan offered by Senator Kennedy; a
vast new expansion of Medicare, as proposed by Senator Javits; or
one of the "milder" proposals for government health financing—
the American patient will pay a high price in terms of the lower
standards of medical care he can expect to receive for himself and
his family.

To repeat the words of Dr. McNeil, recalling his own days in
England's government health program: "I shudder at the risks the
patients ran under my care."

10. The High Cost of Free Medicine

"Free" health programs are expensive whether from a standpoint of total national expenditures or simply what they cost the individuals who support them. "Free" medicine is so expensive, in fact, that national health programs in France and England have brought those countries to the brink of financial disaster; so expensive that government officials have estimated the average American taxpayer may have to pay up to 80 percent more for his family's health care if a national health insurance program is adopted in this country.

At best, the sick and injured would continue to receive the same quality of care they receive now, but experience indicates the quality will be far worse. What, then, would create such a drastic increase in medical costs?

The answer lies in the nature of the two health system alternatives: private practice on the one hand; a government-financed program on the other.

Under a system of private practice, the patient pays only for the care or service he receives. If he receives 20 minutes of a physician's time, that is what he pays for, regardless of how much service the physician renders to the other patients he sees that day. The customer in a drug store pays only for the number of pills he is given, without concern for how many pills the druggist's other customers are purchasing. The patient pays only for his own time in a hospital, not for the time spent by the other patients.

This is not the case under national health insurance.

Under a program of "free" medical care, such as that advocated by Senator Kennedy, for example, you, as a patient, would not pay your doctor a single dime for his services. You would not pay your pharmacist nor would you pay for any time spent in the hospital. Which, of course, makes the program deceptively attractive.

The hitch is, *somebody* has to pay. The physician must make enough to pay for his office space and equipment and to care for his family—and he must make enough of an income in excess of those basic needs to persuade him to continue doctoring. The same is true of the pharmacist. And somebody must pay for the equipment in the operating room, for the hospital beds, for the salaries of nurses and orderlies.

Under the Kennedy plan, and similar programs for national health insurance, all the bills would be paid by the government. But you and I are the government; under national health insurance, we would pay in our roles as taxpayers, rather than as patients—but we would still pay.

Changing Times magazine, in an article on national health insurance, warned its readers: "One way or another, you'll continue to pay plenty for medical care. Don't be deceived by the maximum *direct* costs . . . 'General revenues' means taxes, too—and those taxes will be paid by you and your employer."

Advocates of national health insurance advertise such programs as providing "free" medical care. When they discuss details, of course, they admit that the program is not "free" (except insofar as *direct* costs are concerned), but still contend that such systems reduce the individual's medical care costs by providing "more efficient" care.

Either way—"free," or simply less expensive—national health insurance would be an attractive package for the average taxpaying citizen (who is also, sometimes, a medical patient). But the truth is, government health programs have consistently been far *more* expensive than private medical care—both for the nation as a whole and for the taxpayers who foot the bills. The patient who is treated under a government health program must pay a sum determined (a) by the costs of the program and (b) by his own income. Therefore, in addition to his own medical expenses, he must pay an

additional amount for (a) persons who require or demand more
medical attention than he does, and (b) persons who have smaller
incomes and thus contribute less to the program.

Paying for the care of persons who require or demand additional
attention does not mean simply that the taxpayer's "contributions"
are increased to care for those few who are unfortunately hard hit
by frequent or lengthy illness or particularly disabling injuries. It
is in the nature of the system that the illusion of free care creates
excessive demand and overuse of both the doctor's time and the
hospital's space and facilities. Whether a person concludes that the
cost of the care is being somehow taken care of by somebody else,
or simply determines that he has already paid for it and should thus
try to get all he can, he is "encouraged" to seek medical advice and
care for the most trivial ailments or imagined hurts and to linger
in hospital or sick bed as long as his fancy desires.

In addition, the taxpayer-patient would have to pay for the massive superstructure of bureaucracy and governmental paperwork
that would be required to oversee the largest Federal program in
the nation's history—one that would cover more than half a million
health care providers, and more than 200 million potential patients.

Before the passage of Medicare, Ralph R. Rooke, speaking in
behalf of the National Association of Retail Druggists, warned:
"The plan would produce an administrative nightmare, with federal officials first working out contracts with 6,000 hospitals, 25,000
nursing homes, 700 visiting nurse groups, and later, should physicians services and out-of-hospital drugs be included, with 208,000
doctors and 55,000 retail pharmacists.

"The paperwork involved in processing claims for the 12 million
beneficiaries of the plan staggers the imagination. An extremely
large force of government workers would undoubtedly be required
to do the job."

Rooke's fears came true. Within five years after it had been
adopted, the nation's Medicare law was an acknowledged failure.
Costs continued to soar as Congress continued to increase the price
the aged had to pay to use the program. Government disbursements for the hospital insurance portion alone had reached more
than $11 billion by 1969, more than 40 percent above the original
estimates. Administrative expenses—the cost of maintaining the
massive health bureaucracy created by the program—totaled nearly

half a billion dollars and had more than doubled in the first five years of the program to almost $150 million for fiscal 1970.

Yet the Medicare program covers only Americans over age 65; national health insurance programs would cover 17 times as many people. Obviously the cost would be many times higher. For example, a full 20 percent of the average Swedish citizen's taxes now go to support that country's national health scheme.

The huge administrative force needed to support as massive a project as national health insurance in this country is almost incalculable. Consider for example that without such an enormous program, or any program comparable to it, administrative expenses for government health programs in 1969 totalled almost $282 million.

Dr. Edward McNeil, the British-trained surgeon who fled that country's medical system to practice in the United States, has experienced the results of a massive government health bureaucracy on a first-hand basis:

"After a year in New York which opened my eyes to the tremendous opportunities here and the advantages of private practice, I returned to England for a time to clear up personal matters and to see if I had been mistaken about the NHS (the British National Health System). I spent a year as Casualty Surgeon in a North Devon hospital in a charming small town from which part of the English fleet sailed to meet the Spanish Armada. My pay ($45 a week) was three times as much as when I was a house surgeon and I was given a nicely furnished apartment, but the bureaucratic administration of the hospital was irksome and wasteful . . .

"Although the hospital was small (less than 200 beds) there was a veritable array of administrative assistants. Before nationalization, there had been a maintenance employee who looked after the heating system, lighting and mechanical appliances, with occasional help from outside private firms. At the time I was there, they had a chief plumber, electrician, heating engineer, and other specialists, all under a chief maintenance officer, all complete with offices, desks and secretaries, and inventory clerk. The hospital secretary also had a secretary. A few miles away was the governing hospital of the area, with a large administrative staff to pass on orders to the hospitals in the group; and, of course, *they* were passing on orders from the Ministry of Health in London."

The same thing happened in this country when the government

attempted to run the large Cook County Hospital in Chicago.

"What happens when politicians try to run a hospital?" asked Frank Blatchford III, a Chicago reporter. His answer: "A tale of patronage, mismanagement, and administrative bumbling . . ."

"A big city political machine runs on patronage," Blatchford wrote, "and the hospital provided thousands of jobs."

Dr. Robert J. Freeark, the hospital's superintendent until he quit in frustration after less than two years, complained: "The budget would call for 50 custodial workers. We could probably have done the job with 10 persons if we had paid them a little more, but it was to the advantage of the politicians to have 50 patronage jobs."

Fearful of the vast cost of the bureaucratic network that would be required to operate a national health insurance program, Hugh H. Ross III, an executive with the Metropolitan Life Insurance Company, wrote in the *Washington Evening Star:*

"While the proponents of nationalized health insurance advance costs as a major incentive for turning the whole program over to the federal government, we should bear in mind the government's poor record as an institution capable of holding down cost. A program as extensive as the one proposed would create a new federal bureaucracy comparable in size to the Defense Department. I am at a loss to understand how we can expect any substantial cost savings, particularly if we look, for example, at the record of the Defense Department."

Examining the effects of administrative red tape on the British medical system, Melchior Palyi, author of *Medical Care and the Welfare State*, wrote:

"From the administrative angle, nationalization raises weighty problems. Bulk-buying was expected to lower the cost of hospital supplies. But governments are poor marketers and the advantage of their buyer's monopoly is canceled by the clumsiness of their maneuvering. British hospitals complain that the poor quality of the "cheap" supplies increases costs . . .

"Under socialism the life of a hospital manager is not easy. There used to be a sort of nationwide competition in economy of management. Now economy is of no avail; the savings disappear into the general trough. Economy is actually discouraged; the more money a management requests, the more it is likely to get, provided it

keeps in step with the others. But they all try to get the most—
which keeps them in step.

"Excessive red tape is the universal complaint. Hospital managers are literally swamped by Ministerial decrees and their legalistic
interpretations. Down to the smallest details of administration, the
question is not to decide on what is best, but to check on the
voluminous files to see what the High Authority has prescribed,
and how to avoid procedural errors. Every professional recommen-
dation has to travel back and forth among overlapping medical
committees, the local Hospital Management Committee, and the
Supervisory Regional Hospital board, 'so that a debate on a particular point may extend over many months.' The 'mountainous addition in work' results in a great increase in the clerical staff. . ."

Soon after the National Health Service was created, the British
Auditor General reported: " . . . of the total hospital expenditures,
9.9 percent goes in doctors' (specialists') salaries, 23.8 percent for
nurses, *and 26.5 percent represents salaries and wages of 'other officers and
employees' including administrative staffs.*"

The bureaucracy of government medicine adds nothing to the
quality of medical care; to the contrary, it creates delay and inefficiency, dangerously impairing the quality of treatment. Yet each
year taxpayers in nations with government health programs pay vast
sums of money to support this unavoidable ingredient of nationalized medicine. Such a high price does government bureaucracy
exact that the *Dallas Morning News* recently commented: "The
biggest item on the middle-class American's budget today is not the
cost of health care . . . The biggest cost is the cost of government . . ."

But the obvious administrative costs of government medical
programs are far from being the entire costly story. There are
other costs that will eat just as heavily into the dwindling pock-
etbooks of the silent majority who put up the money to support
the government's vast expenditures. In an age of inflation, with
government policies rewriting price tags on everything from automobiles to ground beef, control of the inflationary spiral has
become a major obsession of politicians and economists. Yet the
creation of vast new bureaucracies such as that which would be
necessitated by the proposed national health insurance programs
would send the inflationary flames to new heights, adding heavy

new burdens to the taxpayers' sagging shoulders.

Commenting on the danger of such a natural corollary to national health programs, syndicated columnist John Chamberlain warned that "the government, to put Reuther-Kennedy into effect, would have to create an entirely new federal insurance bureaucracy. The inflationary potential in such an approach is . . . a bit frightening."

The cost of bureaucratic regulation will also be felt in higher bills for physician care and hospital stays. Dr. George C. Roche, President of Hillsdale College, cautioned recently that "Hand in hand with lack of price discipline comes the problem of bureaucracy . . . Records grow steadily more complex, forcing steadily more doctors and hospitals to add personnel and equipment to process paperwork. Rest assured that those substantially increased costs are reflected in patient's bills."

Dr. George Graham, a former president of the American Hospital Association, has estimated that in the first few years of Medicare the number of man-hours spent by "administrative and general" employees in hospitals increased by 15 percent. With hospital employees finally being brought up to wage levels commensurate with those in the general community, after years of low-scale salaries, the large increase in non-medical paper-shuffling and form-filling activities has played a significant role in the increased cost of hospitalization. New government health programs such as national health insurance, which would be many times the scope of Medicare, both in coverage and dollar outlay, could conceivably send hospital costs soaring beyond reach in the next decade.

Doctors, too, have had to expand their facilities to meet the growing requirements of the Federal health bureaucracy. One Maryland doctor complains that whereas in 1950 he had only one employee in his office, he now has three—a girl to answer the telephone and work on the more complicated billing necessitated by third-party payment, a second girl to assist in treating patients, and a third just to handle the paperwork (see Chapter 5). The same is true of doctors in all parts of the country.

But this expansion has been necessary to handle the paperwork arising from only two comparatively small government health programs—Medicare (for the aged) and Medicaid (for the indigent). Obviously a national health insurance program, which would cover *all* of the doctor's patients, would require much greater overhead expenses in both equipment and personnel. As the increase in paperwork since 1965 has resulted in higher fees charged by many physicians, the much greater increase resulting from national health insurance would add still more in the years ahead. While these added costs would not be paid directly by the patient, they would be paid in the form of taxes, the only method the government has of obtaining the money it needs to pay the bills it would assume under the program.

The administrative requirements of government medicine would add to costs in another way, too. Late in 1970, a market research firm, R. A. Gosselin and Company, announced the results of a survey of 900 pharmacists taken in April of that year. The study revealed that many had increased prescription prices "ten percent or more" to cover their expenses in processing Medicaid claims; 15 percent of the companies that responded to the survey had increased their drug prices "across the board" because of the Medicaid paperwork requirements.

R. A. Gosselin, president of the survey firm, reported that the average citizen was not only supporting the Medicaid program with his taxes, but was also required to "subsidize" the program by paying more for his own drugs.

But the administrative costs that flow from government health bureaucracies are only a part of the large cost increases that would result from adoption of a national health insurance program. "No one knows what an all-inclusive plan would cost," warned *Medical News Report*, but the figures "would be enormous."

Richard Crossman, speaking as British Social Services Secretary, admitted recently that the cost of government medicine was "fantastically under-estimated" when his country turned to a national health system. And, he warned, the costs are bound to continue rising.

One of the prime factors in the rapid increase of health care costs under government health programs has been what the prestigious Brookings Institution called "the tendency of insured persons to make unnecessary and often unreasonable demands upon the medical care services."

Under the American free enterprise system of medical care, excessive or frivolous demands for medical attention result only in increased medical costs for the person who receives the care; under

a national health insurance program, with all of the nation's taxpayers footing the bill for the program's costs, all would suffer increased taxation. This, in turn, creates an ever-expanding circle, for
if a taxpayer is forced to pay more to support the program, he will
logically conclude that he might as well get all he can out of it, and
will be tempted to increase his own demands for the medical care
for which he is paying.

This increased utilization of medical services takes many forms:
more frequent calls to a physician's office, more frequent hospital
visits, extended hospitalization, stocking up on prescription items,
increased purchases of such items as dental braces and eyeglasses.
Whether a prospective patient considers the cost "free" to him, or
simply decides he might as well take advantage of the care he has
already paid for, the demand soars—and the taxpayer continues to
pay ever-increasing bills for the health care of all the nation's citizens.

So massive is the increase in health care demands that overutilization of the system often takes a bizarre twist. For example, a recent
report from England reveals that "a growing number of people
with trans-sexual problems" are taking advantage of "free" medical
services to undergo Myra Breckinridge transformations. "In one
London hospital alone," the report said, "seven men have just
changed into women at the taxpayers' expense."

Estimates by the National Health Service indicate that sex-switch
operations will take place at the rate of at least one a month during
the coming year. Each operation requires the services of an expensive team of medical specialists—a consultant psychiatrist, a consultant endocrinologist, two surgeons, and a professor of obstetrics.

"None of those we have treated had any physical basis for thinking they should belong to the opposite sex," said one of the doctors,
"but all had . . . psychological beliefs that they should so be treated
by the rest of society."

Each operation costs the British taxpayers nearly $850.

Under his "free" medical system, the British patient not only
pays for sex changes for his fellow citizens, he also pays large
amounts each year for free wigs. Dr. Patrick Hall-Smith, a consultant dermatologist at Royal Sussex Hospital, recently reported on a
survey that revealed that free wigs, demanded by elderly women
who are going thin on top, are costing the National Health Service,

and consequently the taxpapers, more than a million pounds a year (one pound equals approximately $2.40). According to a report in London's *Medical News Tribune*, the women arrive at British outpatient clinics insisting on their "rights." More often than not they leave with two free wigs, both paid for by the taxpayers.

Joan Hobson, a British reporter, wrote recently that "the attitude of the British public to medical care has become quite illogical" as a result of the popular belief that medical care is either free or has already been paid for. She related how Dr. Elizabeth Brown, a London GP, told a medical conference recently that one of her women patients had been demanding every possible benefit under the NHS so she could afford to set aside money for a private operation to have the ridges and dimples removed from her abdomen (one of the procedures *not* covered by government medicine) —so she could wear a bikini. Of course the taxpayers footed the bills for her excessive utilization of the government program while she was saving for her operation. "A Midlands doctor recounted instances of NHS patients demanding beauty aid, brandy and slimming tablets. One woman asked for cotton wool to stuff Christmas toys and a keen gardener said he would like a prescription for two dozen narrow bandages—'ideal for fastening my exhibition dahlias to their stakes.' "

Prescriptions under Britain's free health system are free, too, and women with headaches often join waiting lines outside a doctor's office to collect prescriptions for pain relievers they could purchase directly from a pharmacist. The stock answer to protests that these women are wasting their own time and the doctor's is simply: "But I'm *entitled* to it!" This eagerness to stock up on "free" medicines has led to a dangerous situation. Aneurin Bevan, sponsor of the plan that created the current British national health system, recently expressed horror at what he described as "a ceaseless cascade of medicine pouring down British throats."

The demands created by the availability of "free" or pre-paid medicine in Britain have not only increased costs directly by means of increased utilization, but have also cut sharply into the nation's output of products and services, the lifeblood of the economy. Reports released in 1970 revealed that the national health program encourages large numbers of employees to take time off from work for minor ailments. According to the Office of Health Economics, each insured person in Britain now misses 15 days of work each year on "sick leave," a figure that costs the country heavily in lost production as well as in cash sickness benefits.

Overutilization—overdemand—is not limited to the British system of government medicine. Experience in this country and throughout Europe indicates that it is a natural corollary of national health programs.

"In Sweden and Germany," wrote Donald Drake, a reporter for the *Philadelphia Inquirer*, "patients are kept in expensive hospital beds for excessively long periods—more than twice the U.S. average . . ."

"Figures show clearly that under socialized medical systems patients spend more time at higher costs in hospitals which are, as a result, overcrowded and difficult to enter . . ." wrote Allan C. Brownfeld, a Washington reporter.

Germany offers a good case in point. Patients treated under Germany's national health insurance program have an average hospital stay of approximately 24 days, three to four times as long as the average stay in the United States. And, of course, it is the German taxpayer who must bear the brunt of the high costs that result from the extended hospitalizations. Germany has no hospital-bed shortage in terms of concrete ratios between population and facilities, but the country's hospitals are continually overcrowded. With the government—that mysterious supplier of unlimited funds —paying the bills, the patient is under no compulsion to leave the hospital any earlier than necessary. Since their patients are under no increased financial burden as a result of the hospitalization, doctors are insensitive to the possibility of cutting down the program's costs by shortening the hospital stays.

Dr. Klaus Rentzsch, a German specialist who has compared his country's medical system with the American system (Chapter 9), reported on the drawbacks to the German program (national health insurance) in a major article in *Private Practice* magazine. Under Germany's form of national health insurance, Dr. Rentzsch wrote, every employee and industrial worker is taxed about 10 percent of his income for health care, with half of the tax paid by the worker and the other half paid by the employer. The insurance covers payment for all medical care, and the employer is required to pay full wages for the first six weeks of an illness—one of the extensions that American sponsors of government health programs may have in mind, judging from remarks by Senator Kennedy that his proposed national health insurance plan is intended not as a final program but as a step toward a more expansive system.

"All medical care is provided by the government, without any direct payment by the patient himself, " Dr. Rentzsch wrote. "Nobody can say how many millions of dollars are wasted this way every year.

"According to our social insurance statistics, tonsillitis caused the average patient to be laid up for 21 days in 1927—and in 1967. In those 40 years therapy developed from aspirin to sulfonamides to penicillin and the other antibiotics. Every medical progress shortened the process of tonsillitis. But not one day was cut off the time the average patient was out of work. This may show what happens when all the risk of a sickness . . . is completely covered. The will of the patient to take up his work as soon as possible is paralyzed . . . The situation is comparable in every country with a total medical program such as ours . . .

"The general feeling is, 'I have paid my contribution to the insurance. Now I am sick. It's the doctor's task to repair my health . . . My only interest is to get as much medical care and drugs as possible, without pay, of course.' "

Costly overutilization is a natural result when the patient's payment is separated from the actual use of the services or facilities.

In a discussion with Wilbur Cohen, former Secretary of Health, Education and Welfare, and an original promoter of the American Medicare program, Dr. Louis R. Zako, President of Detroit's Wayne County Academy of General Practice, asked what could be done to control the costs of the Medicare and Medicaid programs, which "have produced major . . . problems for the consumer."

"I am not too optim stic about solving the problem of costs," Cohen admitted, explaining that "if we have more people getting more care, with more demands on the system, naturally prices will continue to rise."

Turning to the problem of controlling hospital utilization, Dr. Zako complained ". . . it seems to those of us who are in the practice of medicine that most of the pressures for overutilization come not from our colleagues, but from patients . . . We . . . find that patients and their relatives find it more convenient to stay in the hospital until the weekend. There are tremendous pressures on physicians who are resisting these kinds of approaches daily—so much so that we feel frustrated in our attempts to control utilization."

Indeed, experience in this country and in Europe indicates that utilization control is futile under government health programs. Excessive demand for treatment is a natural result of the system. As we noted in Chapter 7, the Kaiser Permanente health program in California offers a good domestic example.

Dr. George E. Shambaugh, Jr., a Professor of Otolaryngology at Northwestern University, reports that in Veterans Administration hospitals a fenestration operation required an average of eight weeks of hospitalization, compared to eight days in a private hospital. "One reason," reported Dr. Shambaugh, "is that the patient, with all his bills paid for him, lacks any incentive to leave the hospital as soon as he is able to."

Representatives of the American Association of Councils of Medical Staffs presented similar findings in testimony before the Senate Finance Committee on September 16, 1970. Using official figures released in *Hospitals* magazine, the council spokesmen compared average hospital stays in seven private New Orleans hospitals with the average stays in the city's two government hospitals.

In the private hospitals, in which most patients pay their own bills, either directly or through private insurance, the length of stay ranged from 6.1 days to 10.4 days, with an average of 8.11. In contrast, the length of stay in the U.S. Public Health Service hospital was nearly 18 days and the average stay in the New Orleans Veterans Administration hospital was 22 days. As a result, even though the per diem charge in the government hospitals was lower (an average of $50.80 per day, compared with an average of $65.57 in the private hospitals), the total cost of the hospital stay was considerably lower in the private hospitals. (The cost per stay in the private hospitals ranged from $392 to $648, with an average of $527; the average cost in the Public Health Service hospital was $922, a total of $274 more than the most expensive private hospital and $395 more than the private-hospital average; the cost per stay in the VA hospital was even more expensive—$1,093 or $445 more than the most expensive private hospital and more than double the cost of the private-hospital average.)

It is not difficult to foresee that hospital costs would soar if the entire nation were suddenly covered with the same "free" medical service that is offered in the government hospitals in New Orleans. Excessive demands and overutilization would create staggering hospital bills that we would pay in the form of higher and higher taxes.

We can get some idea of the increased costs of health care that would result from the widespread overutilization that would follow a national health insurance program: It has been estimated that more than one billion dollars a year could be saved if the average length of stay in the nation's hospitals were reduced by only one day. The opposite conclusion would be equally valid—that the *addition* of one extra day to the average hospital stay would *cost* one billion more dollars a year.

A brief review will indicate what additional expenses might follow a program of national health insurance:

—*One* extra day on the average hospital stay might cost *one* billion extra dollars a year.

—In Germany, under a program of national health insurance, the average hospital stay is approximately *16* days longer than in the United States.

—In the VA hospitals studied by Dr. Shambaugh, the average hospital stay for a fenestration operation was *48* days longer than in private hospitals.

—In New Orleans, the average hospital stay in "free" government hospitals ranged from *9* to *13* days more than in private hospitals.

Results of California's first four years of experience with the Medicaid program indicate that the overuse of medical services under government programs may be even worse than indicated by the extended length of hospital stays.

Medicaid is a state-administered program of medical services for the indigent, with the state paying half the costs and the Federal Government paying the other half. In 1966-67, the first year of the program's operation in California (where it is known as Medi-Cal), there were 97 claims filed for every 100 persons on the Medi-Cal rolls. By 1969-70, the number of claims had risen to 141 for every 100 persons.

"Medi-Cal services are being overused—a better word is abused —simply because they are "free," complained the *San Francisco Examiner.*

The cost of the program rose from $600 million in 1967 to more than $1.2 billion in 1970. In 1967 it provided free health care to one of every 15 Californians; in 1970 one of every eight Californians was receiving Medi-Cal payments.

The overuse caused by government programs was clearly evident in the Medi-Cal experience. In 1970, the average cost for Medi-Cal health care was $517 *per recipient*, compared with figures released by the Bureau of Labor Statistics that indicate an annual cost of between $540 and $565 for the average American *family of four*.

"[Medi-Cal] has become a monster devouring the state's dollar resources," said the *Examiner*. "The system could bankrupt the state government . . ."

Eli Ginzberg, Professor of Economics at Columbia University, in a paper presented at the Centennial Celebration of New York City's Mount Sinai Hospital, cautioned: "The only real control over costs is to keep the amount of medical services within bounds; to be sure that essential needs are met but that medical services do not expand beyond."

But expansion is the natural course of government health programs, through administrative bureaucracy, through excessive demand, through overuse of facilities.

The *New York Times*, reviewing a book on American medical care, commented:

"The most fascinating side of the discussion is the impersonal way in which hospitals, bureaucracy and cost expand—almost as if by a law of nature. It is fascinating to see, for example, how the presence of Blue Cross has helped bring about the high costs of treatment that it was organized to prevent. The very fact that it was there to provide a steady flow of money for new machines and new procedures gave the green light to hospitals that might otherwise have been more cautious. It wasn't a case of skulduggery, but of unaccountability . . . Various government plans, Medicare and Medicaid, have abetted this trend."

Government health programs spend vast amounts of money— and it's your money. It may, in fact, be many hundreds of dollars of your money—and billions of dollars of your nation's money.

Some comparisons may be helpful:

According to the *Congressional Record*, total Federal appropriations for medical and health care in fiscal 1969 totaled less than $17 billion.

The Social Security Administration has estimated that if reimbursements were made according to the standards followed in the Medicare program—that is, paying physicians, dentists and other participating health care "providers" reasonable costs and charges —the program proposed by Senator Kennedy would cost approximately 77 billion dollars. This would be more than four and one-half times as much as the total 1969 expenditures for the Hill-Burton hospital construction program; the Food and Drug Administration and all the health programs provided by the Department of Health, Education and Welfare (including Medicare); the Department of Defense; the Veterans' Administration; the Office of Economic Opportunity; the National Aeronautics and Space Administration; the Peace Corps; and 15 other departments and agencies.

And it is important to remember that cost estimates for government programs are generally notoriously low. For example, even *The New Republic*, a liberal publication that has supported the concept of government health programs, admitted in a recent article by health-affairs writer Mel Schechter that Medicare alone, without any changes or additions, requires an immediate tax increase to avoid a projected 25-year deficit of $236 billion in hospital-related benefits—an overrun of 100 percent.

Professor Myers, drawing on his experience as chief actuary of the Social Security Administration, gave a striking example of the discrepancies between cost estimates and actual expenditures in an article entitled "How Did Medicare Costs Compare With Original Estimates?" in *Private Practice* magazine.

"The original estimate of disbursements for HI [hospital insurance] benefit payments and administration expenses for insured persons for the period of July, 1966, through June, 1969, was $7,142 million," he noted.

"These figures are shown on a calendar year basis in the Actuarial Cost Report issued by the House Ways and Means Committee on July 30, 1965. The actual disbursements for HI benefit payments and administrative expenses for this period (on a 'cash' basis, representing actual payments from the trust fund) were $11,236 million, or 41.1 percent higher than the original estimate . . .

"In summary then, the original actuarial cost estimates were definitely too low, as contrasted with the actual experience."

The runaway costs of the Medicare program in this country are not the only example of rapid cost escalation. The Saxon Foundation, in a booklet entitled "British National Health Service—A Lesson for America," reported that England's NHS expenditures increased more than three-fold (from 479 million pounds to more than 1.5 billion pounds) during the years 1950–1968, a period when the total population covered by the NHS was increasing only 10 percent (from 50 million to 55 million). On a per capita basis the government's expenditures for the National Health Service increased from 9 pounds, 10 shillings to 28 pounds, 10 shillings during that period.

There is no sign that the high costs borne by national governments to support such health programs are producing any beneficial results:

—In the United States, cries of medical "crisis" have reached their peak after nearly two decades in which federal health appropriations have climbed from $1.7 billion to nearly $17 billion.

—*Life* magazine has reported that Russia's medical system, the most completely socialized in the world, is in many respects a full half-century behind the United States in providing health care to its people.

—Most of Canada's 20 million citizens are covered by a federal program that offers almost unlimited hospital coverage, and citizens of 7 of the nation's 10 provinces are covered by a plan that pays most physician fees; medical costs in Canada have soared.

—The national health insurance program in France has already run up a deficit of $165 million since World War II; the deficit is expected to reach a staggering $1.8 billion by 1975.

Some other comparisons will help illustrate the enormous financial burden that will result if the $77 billion national health insurance program proposed by Senator Kennedy becomes law:

—National health insurance would cost as much as the entire 1970 U.S. budget for military defense.

—National health insurance would cost 25 times as much as the 1970 budget for the conduct of foreign affairs.

—National health insurance would cost as much as the 1970 budgets for space research and technology, agriculture, housing and community development, education and health and welfare *combined.*

—National health insurance would cost an amount equal to well over one-third of the total United States budget for 1970.

Yet there is distinct disadvantage to talking of such costs in incomprehensible terms, such as multiple billions of dollars. A far more striking comparison can be derived from a review of what national health insurance will cost us as taxpayers, for regardless of who signs the checks, we will put the money in the account.

"The federal budget is a mighty personal thing," reminded the prestigious *Kiplinger Washington Letter* recently. "It's *your* money that's being spent."

The *Dallas Morning News* said somewhat the same thing: "As middle Americans, we delude ourselves if we accept the unspoken suggestion that a compulsory health plan can somehow, some way pass those high medical bills on to somebody else.

"Middle Americans can pay their medical bills by paying the doctor, by paying private insurance premiums, or by paying higher taxes to support socialized medicine—but they must pay them in some form if they are to get the care."

If it is our money that is being spent, how much will national health insurance cost *us?*

". . . If national health insurance is successfully enacted," warned the *Indianapolis Star*, ". . . it will mean that quite soon millions of wage earners, their employers matching them, can look forward to topping the $1,000 a year mark in Social Security taxes alone—and this before they have even begun to pay their 'regular taxes.'" The *Star's* frightening prediction is confirmed by Professor Myers in an article entitled "The Cost Effects of the Kennedy-Reuther Proposal."

According to the original Kennedy plan introduced in 1970, national health insurance would be financed by employer payroll taxes (providing 39 percent of the program's income), direct withholding taxes on individuals (about 21 percent) and general Federal revenues (about 40 percent). Although the individual must also pay for the taxes on his employer (either through lower salaries, reduced fringe benefits, or, as a consumer, through higher prices), it is difficult to calculate the actual individual expense through that indirect tax route. Professor Myers therefore bases his calculations of individual cost on only the direct withholding tax and the individual's share of the 40 percent to be taken from general revenues. "First," Myers points out, "we recognize that the government subsidy . . . must be paid by the taxpayers. It just does not represent money that comes down from Heaven or from Santa Claus; advocates of national health insurance include only the direct withholding tax paid by the individual employee in calculating individual costs of the program, overlooking the fact that the individual also pays the taxes that provide the 'general revenues.'

"For calendar year 1974, the first full calendar year of operation," Professor Myers continues, "I estimate that the income to the system established by the proposal will amount to about $57 billion . . .

"Let us consider next what the tax burden of $57 billion in 1974 means to an individual . . . The $57 billion represents an average payment of about $265 per year from each person in the United States. It can be expressed as an average annual payment of about $660 from each worker in the population . . . Moreover, these amounts would be about one-third higher if the cost estimated by the Social Security Administration were met."

In comparison, as was pointed out in Chapter 5, the average American enjoys quite a bargain in health care under the current medical system. According to the Bureau of Labor Statistics, the average middle-income family of four in this country pays approximately $543 a year for all health care, including hospitalization and surgical insurance premiums, doctor's visits, dental care, eye care and eye glasses, prescription and over-the-counter drugs. This amounts to about seven percent of what the average middle income family spends during the year for goods and services. This figure ($543 for a family of four) comes to only $135.75 per person, but the total may not be valid for purposes of comparison, since the average family of four will usually include two minor children with relatively small health maintenance bills, and no aged persons, with higher health care costs. A more reliable estimate of health care costs per individual may be determined from Social Security Administration statistics on total per capita private expenditures for health services. That figure, in 1968, was $162.65; the figure for 1970, reported on page 5 of the *Social Security Bulletin* for January, 1971, indicated an increase to $172.36.

It has been urged that comparisons between the Kennedy program and current expenditures be based on *total* (public and private) per capita spending (about $277 per year), since Kennedy's Health Security Act would replace a number of current government health programs, including Medicare and Medicaid. That figure, however, does not present an accurate picture of what it actually costs the average American to stay well under private-enterprise medicine. Part of the Medicare income is derived from special taxes on the elderly, and all of the program's benefits go to the elderly. All Medicaid benefits go to the indigent. Both are programs that provide no benefits to the average working man and his family. It would be inaccurate to take all government health spending—much of which is of no benefit to the average individual —and use that figure as an indicator of what it currently costs him to keep well.

Using the latest government figures for private per capita spending we can get a good idea of the actual added cost of national health insurance. The average American had a 1970 health care cost of $172. Under national health insurance the cost would be $265—nearly 75 percent more. The average worker in the United States now pays approximately $430 per year for health care; under national health insurance the average worker would pay $880 per year—more than twice as much. The average American family of four now pays approximately $540 a year for health care; according to the Department of Health, Education and Welfare, the tax bill to support the Kennedy program would cost the same family nearly $1,300 a year.

Government health programs are invariably expensive. Medicare is costly and getting more so. Medicaid is driving state health programs to the brink of bankruptcy. Now members of Congress are proposing a host of vast new programs, one of which (the Kennedy bill) would be the most expensive single program legislated in the history of the United States.

If Congress continues to enact government health programs, much of our income may soon be diverted just to meet the staggering costs of staying well.

11. Has Your Mother Outlived Her Usefulness?

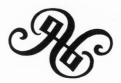

"The National Health Service would have to take greater responsibility for population planning—which would include administration of a program of 'voluntary euthanasia' for the unproductive and incompetent elderly." It would have to "enforce a program of compulsory contraception upon all adolescents, who would later in life have to apply to the Service for permission to produce children. It would then be the job of the National Health Service to evaluate the genetic qualities of prospective parents before granting clearance to beget."

This frightening picture, drawn by Professor Theodore Roszak of the University of California, seems almost surrealistic, an imaginary scene from the depths of science fiction. But there was nothing fictional about recent statements by Dr. Eliot Slater, editor of the *British Journal of Psychiatry,* and Professor Glanville Williams, both of whom have recently presented the arguments for euthanasia—mercy killing—to ease the burden on the government health program in Great Britain.

Even if the elderly do retain their physical vigor, argued Dr. Slater, they suffer from the *defect* of an innate conservatism. "Just as in the mechanical world, advances occur most rapidly where new models are being constantly produced, with consequent rapid obsolescence of the old, so too it is in the world of nature."

Professor Williams, speaking before a nationwide television audience, stated that although the "problem" has not yet reached the point "that would warrant an effort being made to change the traditional attitudes towards the sanctity of life of the aged," the time may come "that as the problem becomes more acute it will itself cause a reversal of generally accepted values."

In June, 1968, the British Broadcasting Corporation aired a special documentary on euthanasia, to consider some of the "forward thinking" among the nation's health experts as they plan the future responsibilities of Britain's national health program. In 1969, a voluntary euthanasia bill was introduced in the House of Lords. The bill would permit the British government to put an elderly patient to death if the patient consented. It is frightening to contemplate the elderly—often weak, in pain, depressed, reminded of their uselessness and of the burden they impose on their relatives and the state—wearily nodding approval to their own execution. So shocking is the movement in Britain that Lord Longford, leader of the House of Lords, warned "the execution time of the old people may not be so far off."

The *London Times* editorially condemned the bill. Pointing to the British abortion law, which has now been expanded to the point that a fetus may be destroyed if its birth would impose on the economic welfare of a family's earlier children, the *Times* warned that "euthanasia once legally admitted would be similarly expanded." Mercy killing of the aged and infirm could easily be expanded to include the "putting to sleep" of other persons no longer useful to society.

How does a society reach a stage where its political leaders can debate eliminating persons who are no longer "useful"? The first step is to surrender control of that individual's life to the government. To put society in charge of your mother's well-being.

That is essentially what will result if the United States enacts a system of national health insurance. Euthanasia is not a part of any of the bills being discussed, but neither was it a part of the national health system that Britain adopted in 1948. Now, however, that government has found it cannot cope with the costs of guaranteeing the health care of all its citizens. No new hospitals were built in Britain for years; there are long waiting lines for hospital admission, and government investigators have angrily condemned the sorry condition of medical facilities. The British government *must* cut costs. Its choices are simple: (a) admit that it is not the government's role to care for the health of the people, or (b) continue to operate the national health system and seek drastic means to reduce costs —such as euthanasia.

In any massive program of government health insurance, manned by armies of bureaucrats, there is an ever-present danger that the distinctly individual human being who is your mother, or your grandfather, may become merely a non-productive figure on a hospital's daily bed chart. Eccentricities and obstinate clinging to "the way we used to do things" will become merely "defects of an innate conservatism." This problem is not unique to Britain. It is part of any system of compulsory national health insurance. Dr. Klaus Rentzsch, who practices under national health insurance in Germany, speaks from experience:

"The more social security is guaranteed by the government, the greater becomes the control over social behavior. One danger of a social security system guaranteed by the state is that personal freedom may be limited because the institution that has to pay for all risks of health may demand that members avoid circumstances which may be a risk to health . . .

"A system that gives free medical care . . . will, of course, try to keep things under control. But control in medicine is a bad thing. Such controls limit the doctor's freedom, his therapy, and even regulate how long a patient stays away from work. All systems of national health insurance believe in this control."

It is obvious that if the United States adopts broad new programs of state-directed health care, the American citizen may pay a high price for them—in the form of new incursions on his privacy and freedoms. Limitations on individual freedom are an integral part of government intrusion into any area of the private sector. As private services, including health care, are re-oriented from traditional person-to-person relationships to a new mass basis, using modern assembly-line techniques, there is an inevitable diminishing of concern for the human individual who is most affected by the new system.

Advocates of government regulation invariably claim to promote their controls in the interests of The People. Their advocacy is hailed as "social awareness." Social awareness, however, is a term used to indicate concern for the well-being of the society. And society is nothing more than a composite of individual beings. There can be no "well-being" for a society unless there is also well-being for its individual members.

Those who seek increased government regulations of medicine —like those who seek a more powerful state in any area of life— express an empty concern, for their concern is solely for The People, without a corresponding interest in the well-being of the individual person. They visualize the good of The People as an abstract concept, or as a statistical mass, without a corresponding concern for the person as a patient in need of a physician he can trust; without a concern for the person as a distinctly individual, sometimes eccentric, sometimes frightened, sometimes lonely, always hopeful, being imbued with very real, and very *personal* needs.

Emerson wrote: "Do not say things. What you are stands over you the while, and thunders so that I cannot hear what you say to the contrary." So it is with those who urge government control of medicine or the establishment of massive, depersonalized health care centers, all the while proclaiming they do so in dedication to the welfare of The People. One is put in mind of Rusanov, the ailing bureaucrat in Aleksandr Solzhenitsyn's novel *Cancer Ward:* "The Rusanovs loved the People, their great People. They served the People and were ready to give their lives for the People. But as the years went by they found themselves less and less able to tolerate actual human beings . . ."

It is this alleged love for The People, this vague proclamation that the pursuit of power is really for the benefit of The People, that wins to the liberal cause many of its idealistic adherents. Yet it is the concurrent lack of concern for the sole individual—the taxpayer, the patient, the person in need of counsel and comfort—that enables a society to come to a point, as it has in Britain, where self-appointed planners can debate, in deadly seriousness, the possibility that it may become necessary to eliminate non-productive or non-useful people for the good of The People.

Government health programs pose other dangers to personal freedom, too—not as dramatic as the recent spate of mercy killing proposals, but of more immediate danger. National medical systems generally disrupt the private-care system of free-enterprise medicine and replace individual care with depersonalized screening systems much like a garage's standarized used-car checkup. Donald C. Drake, a reporter for the *Philadelphia Inquirer,* recently reported on an extensive study of health-care systems in European countries: "None of the European systems studied offered substantial incentives to do a superior job," he wrote. "In England it is traditional for a general practitioner to swiftly send a patient off to the hospital if his care requires anything more than superficial treatment."

The American citizen of the 1960s provided for his own health insurance protection. By the end of the decade, more than 80 percent of all Americans were covered by one or more private insurance policies that enabled them to buy top-quality medical care from whichever private practitioner they preferred. The same situation existed in Sweden prior to the initiation of that country's government health program. At the time Swedish medicine was nationalized, the 70 percent of Swedish citizens who carried private insurance were forced into a compulsory government-administered system to provide for the 30 percent who had not purchased private protection. As a result, there are few private physicians remaining in Sweden. Of the 8,500 doctors in the country, only 1,200 are in private practice—25 percent of them more than 70 years old. Only 30 percent of Swedish patients are cared for by private doctors. Almost all Swedish citizens have been forced to accept government care; today hospitals in that country are overcrowded, with long waiting lists. Patients may have to wait as much as six months for minor operations. Nursing homes and extended-care facilities are understaffed and badly overcrowded, with waiting lists sometimes reaching 2,000. Yet there is very little the Swedish citizen can do about his plight. Freedom of choice has been virtually eliminated in all matters concerning health care.

A similar situation exists in England where two million British citizens, with little freedom of choice available under the National Health Service, have opted to join private health insurance plans —although such a move means they must pay double for their insurance protection, once in the form of premiums to the private companies, and again in the tax bites taken by the government to support its increasingly expensive medical program (see Chapter 9). It is not easy for Britons to avoid the inadequate care offered by the NHS. While some freedom of choice is made available by the shelling out of private insurance premiums, the government has recently been reducing the number of hospital beds available for private patients in an attempt to force the British to remain participants in the nation's failing health experiment.

There is little question that the average citizen feels strongly about the desirability of maintaining a personal relationship with his doctor. A Minnesota physician, Dr. Robert T. Kelly, recently reported on the results of a comprehensive health plan set up to care for employees of the Blandin Paper Company of Grand Rapids, Minn., and the employees of the Itsaca County government. When the plan began, in 1958, approximately 3,100 families were enrolled; by 1963, the program had 7,814 family contracts, covering more than 22,000 people. By 1968, the United Steelworkers became interested in the plan.

Members of the union had been offered supplemental coverage previously through a union contract with Blue Cross and Blue Shield that provided for pre-paid care, without free choice of physician. Approximately 60 percent of the eligible employees had opted to join the plan. When Blue Shield, through the Blandin-Itsaca County plan, offered free choice of physician, nearly 95 percent of the union's members signed up. When members were given a choice between a pre-paid plan with free choice of physician and one with a closed panel approach (in which the facility handles physician assignments), approximately 90 percent chose the plan that offered the patient the right to choose his own physician, Dr. Kelly said.

Obviously, the patient feels strongly about his freedom to choose which doctor will examine and treat him. Yet freedom is not one of the benefits held out by the advocates of government health programs.

In his book *Men, Money & Medicine,* Eli Ginzberg warned that the relative success of military medical care offers few lessons for peacetime, when physicians and nurses are free to work when and how they prefer, and patients are free to seek care wherever they choose. "A 'rationalized' system of medical care requires control over both the purveyors of service and those who seek treatment," he warned.

In a report released by the The Brookings Institution, George W. Bachman and Lewis Meriam concluded that national health insurance "would inject the government into the relationship between practitioner and patient.

"A real danger exists that government actions would impair that relationship and hence the quality of medical care," they wrote.

Wilbur Cohen, former Secretary of Health, Education and Welfare and a prime architect of government health plans, has publicly recognized the need for freedom of choice. "I don't believe in a mandatory decision by government as to the form of organization that the individual physician or consumer should have available," Cohen has said. Yet as the campaign for government medicine picks up tempo, the risk of diminished freedoms increases. So little attention is given to personal freedoms, during this quest for government medicine, that Utah's Wallace Bennett, generally regarded as a moderately conservative member of the U.S. Senate, introduced in late 1970 an amazing addition to the proposed Social Security Amendments.

Bennett's bill, Amendment No. 851 to HR 17550, would have established a system creating so-called Professional Standards Review Organizations, appointed by the Secretary of Health, Education and Welfare, with authority to (a) determine in advance whether or not a patient could be admitted to a hospital, (b) determine how long the patient could remain in a hospital, and (c) give or withhold approval for long-term, non-hospital treatment. Although the entire set of proposed Social Security Amendments failed to clear the end-of-session Congressional logjam, the implications of Bennett's amendment are frightening. Ostensibly, county medical societies would have been given first priority as PSRO committees—provided they agreed to comply with the Bennett law and HEW directives. But one of the provisions in Bennett's amendment called for mandatory release of committee records to the government, a direct violation of medical ethics that would have forced many medical organizations to refuse the task. Refusal would have permitted HEW to appoint compliant committees of laymen to determine in advance whether or not a physician could admit his patient to a hospital.

As in most government programs, efficiency and cost-cutting were the prime motives behind Bennett's proposed amendment. Like the quality of care he would receive, the patient's freedom of choice simply does not enter into the consideration. Although Bennett's bill would have applied initially only to patients making use of government funds, this would have immediately included all Medicare and Medicaid recipients and all patients in VA and Public Health Service hospitals. If national health insurance were to become law, Senator Bennett's frightening amendment would have applied to all Americans.

Lack of privacy is a major complaint under government medical programs. Just as Senator Bennett's proposal would have required PSRO boards to make medical files available to the government, British doctors, writes Melchior Palyi, are required to "keep extensive files and open them at the request of the authorities."

In France, writes Joan Hobson, "workers complain that a swift examination watched by perhaps 50 other people is . . . embarrassing."

Though none of the bills proposed in the United States yet contemplate mercy killings of the elderly, crippled or unproductive, other losses of freedom are definitely imminent:

—*Loss of freedom to choose a doctor.* Both the Kennedy plan and the Nixon plan would initiate major efforts to redirect the American patient into pre-payment group plans (called Health Maintenance Organizations by the Nixon administration, which has publicly stated that it would like to see 90 percent of the U.S. public treated by such a system by the end of this decade).

—*Loss of privacy.* The Bennett amendment, which would have forced the opening of medical records to government inspection, portends a rapid deterioration of doctor-patient confidentiality should the U.S. adopt a national health program.

Government programs have already opened medical records which have long been held inviolate. In late 1968 and early 1969, New York City doctors battled with Health Commissioner Edward O'Rourke over the city government's insistence on inspecting confidential medical records of patients receiving Medicaid funds. "I would not open my records . . . I don't have the right to do it," argued Dr. Samuel Wagreich, a respected general practitioner with an office near Yankee Stadium. "I believe it is an infringement of the private, personal relationship between myself and my patient," he said. "Why should a patient have his personal rights to privacy abrogated because he is indigent? Why should his records be exposed to an inspection agent merely because he is poor?"

The threat to patient privacy was spotlighted again early in 1971 when attorneys for HEW intermediaries demanded the right to inspect confidential patient records before reimbursing hospitals for Medicare-covered treatment.

The story, discussed briefly in Chapter 1, came to light when St. Joseph Hospital in Thibodaux, Louisiana, refused to provide Louisiana Blue Cross with confidential records of patients who had applied for Medicare benefit payments. St. Joseph admitted the need for verification of treatment, and had tendered standard admission and billing forms—normal procedure for Medicare reimbursement. Pushing a new attempt to pry into patient privacy, the government insisted that the hospital also open private records, including consultation notes. The hospital refused.

In refusing, St. Joseph rested on sound medical precedent. The Health Insurance Council has held that "certain information"—including the results of psychiatric examination, notes on the patient's personal and family history, etc.—are "not available from the hospital record for release to third parties."

"The information acquired in a doctor-patient relationship is generally considered to be confidential or privileged communication," the Council has said.

Ethics of the American Hospital Association and the American College of Hospital Administrators also demand that the hospital "safeguard confidential information regarding patients . . ." Even the Joint Commission on Accreditation of Hospitals has made the point clear: "The medical record is the property of the hospital and is maintained for the benefit of the patient, the medical staff and the hospital," JCAH stated (Standard III, interpretation, October, 1969). "It is the responsibility of the hospital to safeguard the information against . . . use by unauthorized persons."

Nevertheless, HEW ruled that unless St. Joseph opened its records to government inspection, "whatever services are involved will be treated as unverified and refunds will be obtained." In other words, the hospital would not be paid, or if payment had already been made, the hospital or patient would have been forced to repay the money. "This includes the *entire* medical record," HEW emphasized.

Government officials claim, of course, that such information would be kept confidential in government records. Yet there is a serious question whether such assurances have much meaning. Testifying before the Senate Constitutional Rights Subcommittee early in 1971, HEW Secretary Elliott L. Richardson conceded that his department sometimes makes "confidential" information available to other Federal agencies.

The committee's chairman, Sen. Sam J. Ervin, Jr., warned that government collection of vast amounts of information about individuals poses a grave potential threat to personal privacy and personal freedom. Ervin's concern was echoed by Michigan law professor Arthur Miller, author of *The Assault on Privacy,* who detailed extensive Federal information-gathering activities, widespread interchange of information between Federal agencies, and the relative ease with which such information could fall into private hands.

Yet the Federal insistence mounts. Supporters of government medical programs have always maintained—with a great deal of logic, frankly—that if government is to pay the bills it must have the right to exert stringent controls (a concept long upheld by Federal courts). It is axiomatic that Federal regulation and Federal invasion of privacy will follow in the way of any national health plan; that has been the case with Medicare and Medicaid, and it will be the case with national health insurance.

Such controls are an integral part of government medical-care programs. As the programs expand, the number and extent of those controls will also expand. "Here, as in most other European countries," writes Germany's Dr. Rentzsch, "there is no chance any more to limit . . . these programs (in order) to maintain personal freedoms."

12. The Man in the Middle

Because he bears the brunt of the inevitable decline in medical care, and because he pays the bills, it seems fair to conclude that it is the patient who winds up with the shortest end of the stick under programs of national health insurance. Yet many doctors, especially those who practice under government medical programs, will not likely concede the point. Whereas the patient comes face to face with the grim realities of national health insurance only when he is sick or injured—or at tax time—the doctor, the man in the middle between bureaucrat and patient, lives with the burdens of the system. It is he who must wake up each morning to the frustrations of government medicine.

And the frustrations are many.

It is unnecessary to indulge in wild speculation in order to determine the likely nature of medical practice under expanded programs of government medicine. As Senator Kennedy has pointed out, other nations have set ample precedent. Writing in the British medical journal *GP*, Dr. Denis Cashman expressed the feeling of many family doctors who must practice under the national health service in that country:

"There may be in the National Health Service a family doctor wholly satisfied with his present terms of service, with the nature and content of his work and the demands made upon him by his patients, and with the present arbitrarily reduced rate of pay that he is offered for his job. There may be such a man, but I have yet to meet him. In discussion with doctors all over the country, one gets the impression that bitter disillusionment is the general feeling today among family doctors . . ."

Dr. Cashman is not alone in his feelings. During recent years, a growing number of British physicians have taken to public grumbling about the life they lead, the degradation of the profession they have chosen, and the deterioration of the medical care they are able to provide.

One frustrated British doctor, William Pickvance, finally threw in the towel early in 1970, after eight years of attempting to work within the British medical system. "The Health Service disillusioned me, and if I was a young man again, knowing what I know now, I would choose otherwise," he said. Dr. Pickvance, who was responsible for the care of some 3,000 British patients, announced that he was leaving the country to enter a practice in the U.S., where he and two other physicians would share the care of 5,000 patients—an average of slightly more than half his patient load in England. By coming to the U.S., Pickvance said, "I hope to realize my full potential."

When he left, Pickvance announced that he had become tired of being a "desk clerk" under the British system. His complaint was a common one. Under programs of government health care financing, citizens rapidly become "patients," flocking to take advantage of supposedly "free" medical service. The result is a virtual flood of trivial complaints and insulting demands that, coupled with the government's own insistence on extensive form-filling and record-keeping, transform British doctors into clerks in a giant nationwide medical department store. Pickvance had come to the United States, in part, because "I think a doctor has more status and his professional skill is held in higher regard in America."

John Sweyn, a British general practitioner, put it more directly: "Our profession is cheapened," he said; "our status is lost."

Although it is possible most American patients are little concerned with the doctor's sense of professional status, the MD, like other professionals (and many other workers) is drawn to his profession largely by non-financial inducements, including recognition by others and an inner sense of accomplishment. Withdrawal of these motivating factors may well lead physicians to think twice about entering a life of 60-hour weeks and the unequaled pressure of medical responsibility. (While it is true that American doctors may not enjoy the option of leaving, as did Dr. Pickvance—because there will be no major nation without a government system of medicine—potential future doctors will still have the option of entering other fields of work.)

There is ample reason for the doctor under government health programs to feel like a "desk clerk" or a "grocer," merely filling orders. One doctor complains that NHS patients come to his office demanding beauty aids, brandy, slimming tablets, cotton wool (to stuff Christmas toys) and bandages (to fasten flowers to their stakes). Time has become a precious commodity in the British medical professional's life. "The paramount need for the general practitioner, at the moment, is time," wrote Walter Davis, editor of a British medical journal. "Time to carry out clinical investigations thoroughly. Time to talk to the patient. Time to relax. Time for family life, since we are all human. Time even for meals. Time —the commodity we need so badly. With fewer doctors, more patients and each requiring an increasing number of medical services, time can only be a steadily diminishing factor. In view of the fate of many of one's colleagues it may even be a matter of life and death."

Indeed it may be a matter of life and death. Overworked British doctors are often forced into early retirement by the rigors of their work and early death is an occupational hazard; recent figures revealed 14 percent of British doctors suffering heart attacks before the age of 50.

Lack of time; overwork; relentless demands by patients for unnecessary attention; persistent bureaucratic pressure for the filling of forms, the stamping, recording, processing, filing of official paperwork. It is the doctors who complain of these burdensome impositions that drain their professional—and even their personal —lives. But it is the patient who suffers most from the natural corollary—less time to spend in diagnosing and treating patients and their illnesses.

Under the National Health System, British doctors are required to sign certificates to enable mothers to obtain cut-rate prices on milk and government maternity benefits, forms certifying that patients are really women (so they will be permitted to buy tax-free corsets), and "sick notes" for employers. The "certificate of incapacity" has rapidly become a joke in Britain. For example, doctors are required personally to certify that they have examined any reported broken limbs, though the applying patient may already have his arm or leg in a plaster cast applied by hospital attendants. So ridiculous is the requirement (a natural extension of bureaucratic obsession with paperwork) that one British MD, Geoffrey Clough, recently wrote of a patient who had suffered amputation of both arms some 30 years ago, but who is still required to furnish a certificate of incapacity each three months in order to obtain disability benefits. Four times each year Dr. Clough must take time out from the care of his other patients to examine the man's amputated arms and certify that they have not grown back.

Other doctors report that they are plagued by patients who habitually take off for a weekend binge and stagger back to their home bases in no shape to face a hard day's work on Monday. Because the government requires medical certificates of inability to work, the weekend bout with the brew becomes both a Monday morning hangover for the citizen and a time-consuming Monday morning interruption for the doctor and his sick patients.

But certificates of incapacity are not the only impositions placed on the doctor and his time by the paper-wielders in government offices. For example, the simple task of vaccinating a family against smallpox prior to an overseas trip becomes a time-consuming hassle. A family of four will require the filling of 12 forms (three each in duplicate). The doctor is then required to examine the four patients again five days later, to see that the inoculations were successful. At that point, he will be allowed to collect $2.40 from the government (60 cents for each patient)—provided he complete and submit forms E.C.N. 682 and E.C. 74 to the government health authorities.

Forms and rubber stamps are as much a part of the doctor's office equipment under a national health program as are his stethoscope and tongue depressors. Every GP is required to keep a supply of more than 22 different forms—forms for permission to add new patients to the rolls, forms to obtain maternity bed space in hospitals, even forms that give expectant mothers official permission to have their babies. As a result of these inevitable corollaries of government medicine, those doctors who remain in Britain's health system are grumbling loudly. Each year, more and more quit the system, quit the country, quit the practice of medicine.

A young woman doctor in the Hampshire area wrote to her Executive Council that she was disillusioned and frustrated by the burden of being a doctor under the government medical system. "I feel I can't stand general practice much longer," Diana Samways wrote. "I qualified to do medicine and the continuous chore of writing certificates day after day is cutting across the very work for which I was trained. If necessary I shall leave clinical medicine altogether."

(American liberals frequently console themselves by imagining that things will be different here. Not so. When five private practitioners in Tell City, Indiana, set up a 24-hour-a-day, seven-day-a-week clinic to serve the townspeople, they had to hire two full-time employees just to process the paperwork required by government programs and private insurance companies.)

The frustrations are compounded by the excessively long working hours of doctors who struggle to keep up with the increasing demand and decreasing supply of medical personnel. Junior doctors employed in Irish hospitals in Dublin, Cork and Galway recently issued strong demands for "shorter," 70-hour, work weeks (they were then working 100 hours a week). The authoritative *Guinness Book of World Records* has reported that the longest work weeks in the world have been put in by doctors in London hospitals who have sometimes spent as much as 136 hours on the job in a seven-day period (an average of more than 19 hours a day).

Admittedly the burden on "junior doctors" (hospital staff men) is heavier than that on the GP in normal practice, but even the typical practitioner will spend a full 12 hours a day at the job, beginning with morning office calls (usually starting about 8 or 8:30 AM) and ending with reports, letters, updating of case histories, and other paperwork after the conclusion of evening visiting hours (usually until 7 PM or later).

The frustrations continue to pile up. Speaking at the annual meeting of the Royal College of Nurses a couple of years ago, Mary Blakeley, the association's president, complained of poor working conditions, low wages, shortages of personnel. "Morale in the nursing profession is lower and dissatisfaction is more rife than it has been within memory," she said. "Unless something is done—and soon—further deterioration is likely to be rapid, with very serious implications to the services of this country. The situation may well become critical and the proper care of patients be imperiled."

Working conditions also provide lengthy lists of frustrations for doctors who are forced to labor in national health vineyards. According to Dr. Joselen Ransome, a London hospital consultant, for example, British hospitals are out of date and inadequate (see Chapter 10). So, too, are the facilities and equipment with which British doctors must work outside of the hospitals. Dr. Edward L. McNeil, a British physician who fled that country's medical system to practice in the United States, wrote in *Private Practice* magazine that he had to work without office X-ray equipment and with "less than meager" laboratory equipment (see Chapter 9).

Dr. George Ostlere, who quit the British health system in 1952 and subsequently became nationally famous as author Richard Gordon, commented on the situation in a 1969 article in *Punch*. "That the doctors keep everyone tolerably healthy with what they've got is the biggest flattery of all," Gordon wrote.

The availability of reports on the British medical system, plus that nation's long experience with government medicine, make it both convenient and logical to concentrate on lessons taken from the English experience. But the problems are part of the picture in any country that has undertaken to provide health care by government edict and through government underfinancing.

Dr. Russell Roth, Speaker of the American Medical Association's House of Delegates and a highly regarded Pennsylvania urologist, recently returned from a tour of the Soviet Union (see Chapter 9). Although Russian officials are careful to conceal sights that they have deemed off-limits to Western eyes, Roth's years of medical background enabled him to make a number of observations about the Soviet health-care system:

—"We hear a great deal about the crowded, shabby, archaic conditions prevailing in some of the older and larger municipal hospitals of our country . . . but even these few American hospitals would compare favorably with the overwhelming bulk of Russian institutions."

—"Even the 400-bed general Rayon hospital in Moscow (a Rayon is a political subdivision of about 80,000 people) had no

urologist on its staff, and the urological consultant, who visits twice
a week, had one small ill-equipped room, bereft of X-ray apparatus,
boasting only three cystoscopes and very little else. Obviously any
patient requiring more than elementary urological study or treatment needs to be referred to an Oblast hospital (a regional or state
hospital collecting from many Rayons)."

—". . . In the Republic of Georgia, at the Institute of Obstetrics,
in Tbilisi, one may see elaborate equipment to record fetal elec-
trocardiograms and fetal electroencephalograms, and many other
fetal functions, even during the process of delivery. On the other
hand, throughout the Soviet Union most deliveries are done by
midwives with only the simplest of equipment."

Roth does not paint a totally bleak picture of medicine in the
Soviet Union. The Soviets have large numbers of doctors and allied
health personnel, highly efficient mobile-care units for cardiac
emergencies, clearly defined systems for gaining entry to the
health-care process. But on the whole, it is not a system many
Americans would care to swap for. And if the frustration is felt by
the patients—if the patients must be satisfied with what they get—
so, too, must the doctors who work in the system as technicians; as
mechanics working on the human machine.

Free enterprise doctors can ease the burden of long hours and
occasional frustrations with the knowledge that their heavy responsibilities are rewarded by commensurate income levels. Not so
under government medical programs. In 1966, the average gross
income of the British physician was approximately $12,000 a year.
From that amount he was required to shell out money for office
space and office equipment, and for nursing and secretarial help—
leaving a "take-home" pay (before taxes) of approximately $6,500
—or less than $550 a month. The situation has improved since, but
British doctors are still grossly underpaid.

As a result, more and more doctors are turning their attention to
the task of securing a decent income, rather than concentrating on
patient care in the knowledge that "the money will take care of
itself." A prime example of this preoccupation with making a living
wage was revealed in mid-1970, when 5,000 members of one
medical society—the Medical Practitioners' Union—voted to join
the ranks of a British labor union, the Association of Scientific,
Technical and Managerial Staffs. "We plan to assist in every way

possible to improve their reward . . . ," union officials promised.

Although government health programs spend more money than do individual citizens in a free-market system, the expenditures are directed largely by political motivations, resulting in inefficiency, overabundance and waste in some areas, and paucity in others. Since there is little potential political return from pay raises to small segments of the society, physicians practicing under such systems invariably end up on the low end of the financial ladder.

British physicians have been conducting a running battle with government officials over pay-increase demands, to the frustration of both the doctors and the impartial mediators who have tried to work out an equitable arrangement for compensation. Pressured by doctors who were working for a ridiculous base of $3 per patient per year, Harold Wilson's Labourite government appointed a special review committee, headed by Lord Kindersley, to suggest a course of official action. The committee's recommendation recognized the extent of the problem: Give all NHS doctors a 30 percent pay increase immediately, to compensate for "too few doctors and dentists doing too much work," the committee urged.

The government took the committee's recommendations under advisement, temporarily, then announced that the full increase would go only to junior (hospital) doctors, with all other NHS doctors to receive an increase of only 15 percent, with any further increases left to the decision of another agency, the Prices & Incomes Board. Lord Kindersley and his colleagues on the review board submitted their resignations. The British Medical Association called an emergency meeting.

"The Review Body was our anchor in the ghastly world in which we work and live," mourned Derek Stevenson, a BMA official.

Protesting doctors went on partial strike (refusing to sign medical certificates of incapacity for work), and the BMA once more polled its members about the possibility of a mass resignation from the NHS—a tactic frequently discussed but never pursued. Baseball fans know that the players never win an argument with the umpire. In Britain, as in all other government health programs, it is the government that wears the blue uniform and makes the decisions. As in baseball, the players inevitably lose. The profession settled for a 15 percent increase.

After the 1970 elections swept the Labor government from

power, British doctors turned hopefully to Conservative Edward Heath—and learned that governments continue in their inexorable ways, though faces may change and nameplates may be rearranged on the desks in Whitehall or in Washington. Richard Crossman, the Labor government's NHS overlord, was replaced by Sir Keith Joseph, who promptly informed British doctors that "full implementation of the Kindersley report could have most damaging economic consequences." The "friendly" Conservative government threw the doctors a sop—another five percent increase—that left them still 10 percent short of the pay hike recommended by the government-appointed review board.

The truth is, implementation of the Kindersley report *would* have created economic difficulties for the government. As Americans have learned, governments seldom restructure priorities or phase out expenditures; instead, they pile new programs on top of old ones, and new expenses on top of old ones. In times of financial hardship, governments talk in terms of higher or lower interest rates, printing or not printing new money, controlling or not controlling wages and prices. The discussion centers around whether or not it shall be made more difficult for the citizen to spend and/or save money; there is seldom discussion of a reduction of government spending.

This is the problem faced by British doctors and by doctors in all government health programs (including the American Medicaid program, in which doctors are frequently reimbursed only a reduced percentage of normal charges). The government cannot give British doctors more money, but it is not because there is no more money; it is because there is no more money if the government continues to spend at least as much as it has been spending for other items.

In June of 1970, the medical profession in Britain removed its sanctions, such as they were, in exchange for the government's pledge periodically to review doctors' pay. Nothing happened. In September, under pressure, the government agreed to a meeting —and then postponed it. The meeting was set again, postponed again. Finally, on October 21, the doctors were notified that the government was considering establishment of three interlocking review boards that would not consider physician pay separately, but would include it in a general review of wages in several professions, a proposal that would be discussed with the doctors in a meeting on November 5. On November 2, three days before the scheduled meeting to discuss the proposal, the review boards were announced.

Joan Hobson, reporting on the new disillusionment, wrote: "It now seems likely that open conflict will again arise between the medical profession and the government."

It does not really seem likely at all. One can only wonder how many times it is possible to recreate an illusion and thus open oneself to repeated disillusionment. For British doctors, the answer seems to be: forever. With no effective sanctions forthcoming from a seemingly helpless medical association, more and more doctors, fed up as individuals, are quitting their practices and fleeing to the United States and other lands.

Dr. Patrick O'Kelly, an assistant radiotherapist at St. Thomas' Hospital in London, left England in 1967 to trade in his $2,400-a-year job for a $24,000 post as a radiotherapy consultant in the United States. But there might have been good economic reasons for Dr. O'Kelly to come to the U.S., even if he had not landed a job at 10 times his immediate salary. A British physician can expect to retire, after some 40 years of service, with an income of approximately $600 a month—in sharp contrast to doctors in free-enterprise systems who earn enough money to enable them to set aside funds for a comfortable retirement income.

In the United States, the average physician can count on income escalation as he gets older, becomes more skilled, and attracts more patients. The British physician, on the other hand, begins his practice with a maximum patient load and, thus, maximum income. Because he is paid a flat fee for all service, his income cannot increase as he matures and becomes more proficient. In fact, in 1969, the seniority pay "bonus" for veteran British MDs was fixed at a meager $480 a year for the first 15 years on the Medical Register, and an additional $480 a year after 25 years.

In Austria, where doctors have been laboring under national health insurance plans since the 1880s, the average family doctor has a pre-tax net income of approximately $5,000, less than the income level of many non-professionals.

Doctors in France are only slightly better off. A recent article in *Paris Match* reported that the average net annual income of doctors practicing under the French health system is approximately $700 a month, with income tax taking one-third of the physician's earnings. When the French medical profession complained that fees had risen by only 15 percent in two decades, the government reluctantly granted doctors a small pay raise, under pressure—and then retaliated by abolishing tax incentives that had previously been given.

An Austrian doctor, quoted anonymously by *Medical Economics*, summed up the frustrations: "This system is pretty tough on us doctors," he said. "It's pretty tough on patients, too."

But frustration and low pay are only symptoms of the "ghastly world" of Dr. Stevenson and his medical colleagues. The disease, itself—the cancer that has sapped the strength of European medicine—is government itself. In a word: control. Regulation is the key to any government medical program. That which a government finances, it inevitably controls. In fact, the United States Supreme Court has long held that government has an obligation to control that which it finances. The result has been both chaotic and dictatorial. Regulation has become regimentation, and both doctor and patient have suffered.

Governments, of course, cannot control. Only people can do that. Only people can write the regulations, interpret them, and enforce them. The result is a vast bureaucracy of government officials, frequently without medical knowledge, charged with the responsibility of determining whether diagnoses were accurate, whether the drug products prescribed were the most effective, whether the course of treatment was proper, whether the doctor made too many or too few visits to the patient's hospital bedside.

Just as the bureaucrat is unable, through lack of knowledge, to regulate properly, he is unlikely, through lack of personal contact with those he regulates, to act either with justice or compassion. Bureaucracy, as Alvin Toffler points out in his book *Future Shock*, is an organizational form suited to automatic, unthinking response to standard-form situations. In Toffler's words, "bureaucracies are well suited to tasks that require masses of moderately educated men to perform routine operations . . ."

Dr. Laurence J. Peter, author of *The Peter Principle*, also saw the limitations of the governmental hierarchy: "Particularly among minor officials with no discretionary powers," he wrote, "one sees an obsessive concern with getting forms filled out correctly, whether the forms serve any useful purpose or not. No deviation, however slight, from the customary routine will be permitted . . . the paperwork is more important than the purpose for which it was originally designed. He (the bureaucrat) no longer sees himself as existing to serve the public; he sees the public as the raw material that serves to maintain him, the forms, the rituals and the hierarchy!''

It is this bureaucracy—the bureaucracy described so aptly by Toffler and Peter, but encountered, probably, by each reader of this book—that dominates the practice of medicine in England, France, Austria, Scandinavia, the Soviet Union and the other nations that have adopted national health programs.

Joan Hobson, writing in the March, 1966, issue of *Kiwanis Magazine*, described the situation this way:

"Since socialized medicine was introduced in the British Isles, doctors have been struggling against terrific odds to make a success of this all-time high in welfare service. But now they are exhausted to the point of being physically incapable of dealing with the work load imposed by over-demanding patients . . . lack of money is not their main grouse. Government directives and restrictions have robbed them of the clinical freedom essential to the practice of good medicine."

Enactment of the National Health Service program transformed the British doctor overnight from entrepreneur to salaried civil servant, and he immediately ran headlong into the full implications of medicine by bureaucratic decree. As soon as the program became law, government-issued British MDs were forbidden to sell their practices. Although technically the practices remained the personal property of the doctors who had purchased or developed them, the government had taken away one of the essential characteristics of private property—the owner's right to enter into a contract to sell his property at a price mutually agreed upon by buyer and seller. Overnight, the value of an individual medical practice plummeted. Whereas physicians had been able to sell their practices for approximately three times a single year's income, they were now forced to sell to the government, which, without competition, set the purchase price at only 1.5 times annual income. (The government was also setting the income, by limiting the number of permitted patients and regulating the doctor's payment for each patient on his list. With a typical doctor's annual income likely to fall slightly under $7,000, the government was able to buy the practice for approximately $10,000. If the same practice, with the same income, were sold on the open market, it might well have brought twice that amount.)

Since every doctor would some day either retire or die, eventually the government would take over every individual practice. Doctors who had purchased practices before the government takeover suddenly found the value of their property cut by half. At one fell swoop, British doctors found themselves out $10,000 or more.

In exchange for this newly decreed right of eminent domain over the doctor's practice, the government agreed to pay "interest" at the low rate of 2.75 percent on the purchase price until the doctor retired, when he would receive the lump sum payment, such as it was.

Of course, doctors who refused to participate in the National Health Service, and retained strictly private practices, could continue to sell their practices on the open market. But the government program had virtually eliminated all private health insurance and had imposed compulsory nationwide taxation to support the NHS, thus leaving few Britons willing to pay private medical fees in addition to the taxes they were forced to pay for "free" care. As a result, private practices survived only in posh resort areas where well-off citizens could afford the double charge. In recent years, as the low quality of government medicine has become widely apparent, there has been a resurgence of private insurance with more and more Britons, even in lower-income levels, willing to pay double for health care. But even today, private practitioners draw from only about four percent of the British population. Thus, private practices are scarce and command such high purchase prices that few doctors can undertake the risk.

Thus it was that the British doctor was introduced to the hazards of practicing under government regulation. There was more to come. Bureaucratic decrees soon placed stringent limitations on the quality of care a doctor could dispense. "The norm" became the standard, and the physician, educated to do his best, found that "the best" consisted of satisfying political, rather than patient, needs.

A government-established Pricing Bureau immediately began to establish form-book guidelines. Average prescription outlays were determined, and the doctor whose prescriptions cost more than the average was likely to find himself reprimanded by government employees, with the "excess cost" of expensive prescription items deducted from his next monthly paycheck. A doctor who continued to prescribe high-cost items found himself subject to fines of as much as $280.

While cost reduction is always desirable, the bureaucrats who administer government health programs frequently overlook the fact that the prime objective of medical care is to restore health in the shortest time possible. To accomplish this goal, doctors must be free to prescribe the *best* treatment possible, or the least expensive treatment *that will do the job.* A cut-rate medicine that does not do the job it is meant to do is expensive at any price. If the patient fails to recover, or if he remains ill and out of work for longer than necessary, because of economies pre-ordained "by the book," by officials unfamiliar with the patient or his illness, then the cost of those economies will be high indeed. Nonetheless, Ministry of Health officials make periodic rounds to impress upon doctors the necessity of prescribing the cheapest drugs available for all patients. In addition, doctors who prescribe effective but non-standard remedies may find the entire cost of the treatment summarily deducted from their pay.

Even in the United States, government officials have moved to impose inflexible guidelines on medical and quasi-medical activities. Three prime examples have made recent headlines:

1.   Bound by rigid Congressional guidelines (the Delaney Amendment), the Food and Drug Administration was forced to order all food products that contained cyclamates (an artificial sweetener) from the market. The Delaney Amendment lays down strict orders for the instant removal of any product that is shown to cause cancer in humans *or animals.* Abbott Laboratories, a leading cyclamate producer, routinely notified FDA officials that large doses of cyclamate additives had produced signs of tumors in laboratory rats. Immediately, the FDA imposed a strict ban on the product, ordering the sale of cyclamate-bearing soft drinks and other food products to be stopped no later than July 1, 1970.

At the time of the ban, neither private nor governmental scientists had uncovered any evidence of cancerous effects in humans. They still have not. What's more, the rats that had developed tumors had been fed such massive doses of cyclamate that it would have been virtually impossible for any human to ingest the additive in similar proportions.

Cyclamates were used primarily as a sugar substitute, thus benefiting Americans of all ages who suffered from obesity (with its attendant danger) and diabetes. Sugars, known to be harmful to both groups, again replaced cyclamates. Because of governmental inflexibility (the FDA had no alternative under the Delaney legislation), a product which had proven harmful only to rats when force-fed massive doses was replaced by a product proven scientifically to be harmful to millions of persons.

2.   Late in 1970, the FDA began making sounds about the possibility of removing so-called "combination" drug products from the market. At the request of the FDA, the National Academy of Sciences-National Research Council, a secretive coterie of academicians, undertook a massive study of drug products to decide whether, in the study group's opinion, the drugs were "effective." The result was a list of some 400 drug products that the NAS-NRC maintained ". . . lack substantial evidence of effectiveness." Many of the products on the list were the "combinations"—fixed-dose mixtures of various ingredients, such as cough suppressants, sedatives, anti-expectorants, pain relievers, etc.—that make up a large percentage of the medicines prescribed each year.

According to the government, pre-established dosages make it difficult to practice good therapeutics (implying that doctors will be too lazy to prescribe doses separately if needed, or to consider possible adverse reactions to some of the combined ingredients).

Combination drugs have long been favored by physicians for several reasons:

(a) They are easy to administer. Patients taking combination drugs containing three ingredients each would have to take three pills instead of one to obtain the same medications separately. Thus, a patient taking a three-medicine combination (for example, an analgesic containing codeine, aspirin and phenobarbital) three times a day would have to take nine pills instead of three.

(b) Decreased chance of medication error. By reducing the number of pills to be taken, doctors reduce the chance of patients taking the wrong pills. For example, whereas a patient might take one combination pill three times a day, drawing the tablet from a bottle of similar tablets, he or she might by mistake take three dosages of codeine, or aspirin, or phenobarbital, rather than one of each. This is especially likely among the elderly who consume much of the nation's drug-product output—and likely to be dangerous if the patient is being treated with antibiotics or similarly potent medications.

(c) Reduced cost. Much of the cost of medicine is in the preparation, rather than in the ingredients themselves; even with multiple ingredients, the cost of one tablet is invariably less expensive than the cost of three, and the cost of three tablets per day is considerably less expensive than the cost of nine. By the middle of 1971, intensive pressure from irate physicians had caused the FDA to back off from its proposed combination-drug restrictions.

3.   A third example of governmental interference with prescribing has surfaced repeatedly in the last few years as the result of intensive efforts to force the enactment of an official Federal drug compendium, similar to the British directory of Ministry-approved medicines. Although the compendium would serve other purposes as well, its most immediate effect would be to promote the prescribing of medications by their generic (non-brand) name. Such an official drug list is part of the Kennedy-sponsored national health insurance bill, and liberal legislators in the U.S. Senate and in a number of states have been pushing in recent years to require doctors to prescribe generically. Already, some states have adopted generic prescribing laws.

The advocates of generic-name prescribing contend that if Drug A contains the same ingredients, in the same amounts, as Drug B, both products are identical. Therefore, by prescribing the drug that is not sold under a widely advertised brand name, the doctor will be giving his patient the same medication for less money.

In the formulation of any complex product, however, there are many variables besides the raw ingredients. Nobody would contend that all automobiles are the same, though each operates on the same mechanical principles and contains essentially the same ingredients in the same arrangements. And almost every housewife has run into the frustrating phenomenon that results when she follows a cake recipe to the letter, adding the ordered ingredients in the specified amounts, only to end up with a sunken top layer, a doughy taste, or a grainy frosting.

Similarly, there is more to producing a drug product than pouring the contents of beaker A into beaker B. There are more than
30 variables, ranging from coating to solidifying agents, that affect
the essential nature of a drug product—how fast it dissolves and
enters the blood stream, how much is excreted, how much remains
in the patient's system, etc. One widely reported recent case illustrated the dangers of assuming that generically equivalent products
are necessarily the same: when X-rays revealed a large abdominal
mass in a seriously ill patient, surgeons investigated and found that
undissolved antacid tablets—low-cost substitutes for a highly regarded antacid product—had impacted in the patient's stomach and
caused a dangerous blockage.

Crawford Morris, a prominent malpractice defense attorney, has
warned that physicians who rely on their knowledge of Drug Product A to prescribe generically, in the belief that all of Product A's
generic equivalents will be therapeutically equivalent, run the risk
of exposing themselves to potential malpractice liability. Yet legislators, looking for the political benefits that will flow from their
identification with a reduction in drug prices, continue to push for
generic prescribing.

In addition to these "prescribing" examples, many doctors now
practicing in the Medicare and Medicaid programs in this country
have come face to face with bureaucratic medicine as clerks for
Social Security Administration intermediaries challenge house
calls, hospital visits, and medications.

As the physician surrenders control of his practice to governmental authorities, he surrenders much of his dignity as well. British MDs frequently complain that patients, who carefully address
their plumbers and mechanics as "mister" and courteously request
their services, are prone to be much more brusque in their dealings
with physicians who have become, in effect, medical handymen.
Unlike physicians in the United States, who serve only their patients (unless the patient is covered by a Federal health program,
such as Medicare and Medicaid), British doctors serve multiple
masters.

"It is said that no man can serve two masters, but under the NHS
the unfortunate doctor is expected to serve three," complains Dr.
W. H. Spoor, a British physician: "(1) the patient . . . (2) the
General Medical Council, which can strike his name off the Medical

Register . . . ; and (3) the Ministry of Health, which can fine him
. . . and, through its local executive councils, can compel a doctor
to accept on his list a patient to whom he objects, as has happened
to me."

Although the medical system in France is not truly socialized
(French doctors are not on salary), the government reimburses
patients for 80 percent of their health-care expenses, and thus exerts
extensive control over medical practice in that country, too. Physicians who practice under the government health system must agree
to abide by a bureaucratically decreed schedule of fees, and abide
by a weighty volume of official regulations. Because controls flow
naturally with the money that finances the program, French doctors
frequently find bureaucrats meddling in the care for which they
provide the funds. One result has been a severe limitation on the
ability of doctors to prescribe the medicines or supplies they feel
necessary.

"We resent the government ordering us to prescribe economically," complained Dr. Louis Amour, in Paris, "but we all try to
obey; even so, the Consular of Medicine sometimes reproaches us
for extravagance."

At times the harassment borders on the ridiculous. A French
medical journal recently reported a case in which a doctor prescribed six rolls of gauze and 12 bandages for an injured patient.
Employees of the Health Ministry, without seeing the patient, determined that the injury needed only half that amount—and forced
the doctor to repay $3 for the extra gauze and bandages.

Perhaps the most striking example of governmental regulation,
however, has taken place much closer to home, in the Canadian
province of Québec. Almost unnoticed by the mass media in the
United States, the Québec government, in late 1970, ordered 4,-
000 striking physicians to perform their services or face stiff fines
and imprisonment. The drastic order was part of a major showdown
between Québec medical specialists and the provinical government
over a law that may eventually have far-reaching implications for
all Canadian and U.S. doctors and their patients.

Québec's Medicare Act became law in mid-July, 1970, and included a stipulation that government payment would be limited to
(1) physicians who participate in Medicare, or (2) patients of physicians who participate in Medicare. The Medicare laws in other

Canadian provinces and in the United States, on the other hand, permit payment either to participating physicians or to eligible patients, regardless of whether their physicians are in the Medicare program. The Québec law, in effect, took away the physician's privilege of "opting out" or refusing to participate in the program.

In the United States, many physicians have enacted Individual Responsibility Programs (IRP), informing their patients that they do not recognize the Federal Government's right to intervene in an essentially personal relationship between physician and patient. Doctors who have followed the IRP formula continue to treat patients on the Medicare rolls, but refuse to fill out government report forms, release patient information to government agencies, or accept Federal payment. Instead, they bill patients directly and let the patients bill the government for reimbursement if they choose. The results are the same for the patient—Medicare pays the bills—but the doctor keeps his independence, maintains the confidentiality of his records, and keeps out of any position where he might be influenced in his treatment by the suggestion of third parties who pay the bills.

The Québec law eliminated the possibility of direct patient billing. If a physician did not participate in Medicare, his Medicare patients would not be paid. To collect their benefits, the patients would have to be treated by physicians who did participate in the program. Doctors who refused to go along with the government thus ran the risk of losing large numbers of patients and significant income. In areas with large numbers of elderly citizens, non-participating physicians faced the danger of being put out of business. As a result, immediately after the legislation was passed, 1,500 members of the Québec Federation of Medical Specialists attended an emergency meeting where they voted, almost unanimously, to fight the law. The federation's president, Dr. Raymond Robillard, a prominent Montreal neurologist, told a news conference that the doctors felt they must "protect the liberties of our profession."

"We reject conscription of doctors in a system of state medicine," Dr. Robillard said. "We are not fighting for privileges, but for our freedom."

As the government moved to implement the law, virtually forcing all physicians to participate in the program, Dr. Robillard led his fellow doctors out on strike. For eight days, 3,000 specialists—

including all surgeons, anesthesiologists, radiologists, pediatricians, and obstetrician-gynecologists in the province—refused to work. Another 1,000, also on strike, remained on duty to provide emergency service at 39 of the province's 250 hospitals. Then the government passed Bill 41, ordering the doctors to work—virtually conscripting 4,000 doctors into government service. To enforce the order, the government levied fines of up to $500 a day for every day a doctor failed to work, and imprisonment of up to a month for every day off the job.

Bill 8 (the Québec Medicare law) is a prime example of government regulation at its worst, forcing physicians to participate in federal health schemes or close their offices. But Bill 41 goes a step further: it forbids doctors the option of closing their offices. It orders them to work.

Government medicine has not yet progressed that far in the United States, though participants in the existing Federal health programs have felt the squeeze of the omnipresent governmental hand on the shoulder. As the inevitable overutilization created by the public belief in "free medicine" creates a strain on health budgets, administrators of Medicare and Medicaid programs have resorted to various schemes to reduce medical fees, including a complicated arrangement based on "payment at X percentile" and determination of "usual, reasonable and customary" fees using charges from previous years, before inflation had boosted physician overhead and cost-of-living expenses. Social Security Amendments proposed in the 1970 session of Congress (HR 17550) would have authorized the government to set fees for Medicare treatment at 75 percent of prevalent physician fees—the first major piece of medical fee-setting legislation introduced in Congress. The bill passed the House but was bottled up in House-Senate Conference and eventually died. It was an ominous sign of things to come.

At the same time, members of Congress were moving quietly to impose extensive new Federal controls in other areas as well. Amendment 851 to the Social Security Act, introduced by Republican Senator Wallace Bennett, of Utah, would have required advance Federal approval of hospital admissions under Medicare, and would have given the government power permanently to exclude physicians from participating in Federal programs. The amendment, which would have created Federal policing agencies known as Professional Standards Review Organizations (PSRO), would have permitted government-appointed committees to supersede physician judgment in determining whether ill patients should be hospitalized, treated in nursing homes, or required to travel daily to hospital out-patient facilities for treatment (see Chapter 11). Concerned doctors warned that placement of such extensive power in the hands of Federal administrators, who would not be directly involved with the patients affected by the regulations, might lead to a dangerous rationing of hospital care in an attempt to hold down mounting Medicare costs.

Under the Bennett proposal, Federal committees, using computerized data without actual patient contact, would have determined not only whether a patient could be hospitalized, but for how long. And if a patient did not respond in the time indicated by national averages, physicians would have to seek approval for extra patient time in the hospital. One provision of the proposal would have authorized the Secretary of Health, Education and Welfare to bar physicians from participating in government programs if they refused to comply with HEW regulations promulgated under the law. In areas with large numbers of elderly or poor citizens, permanent exclusion of physicians from Medicare and Medicaid programs would effectively put them out of practice. Among the provisions with which doctors would have to comply, however, was a requirement that patient records be made available to Federal agents "as the secretary may require"—a demand that would force physicians, if they complied, to violate canons of medical ethics and disregard long-standing legal precedents protecting the confidentiality of doctor-patient communications.

At the time of this writing, the Bennett amendment has been reintroduced, with some changes, but has not yet become law. Regardless of whether the Bennett amendment is passed by Congress, the evidence is clear that the government, even with the limited Federal health programs now on the books, is moving rapidly in the direction of control and regulation. The Bennett amendment was passed by the Senate Finance Committee the first time it was introduced—an ominous warning to physicians and laymen who cling to the hope that somehow things will be different here than in the other major nations that have placed health care responsibilities in the willing hands of government officials.

In nation after nation, physicians today give vocal testimony to the disenchantment that has followed the enactment of government health programs. British MDs, writes Joan Hobson, "are acutely aware they are being exploited. They have become pen-pushers; their work is no longer pure medicine; they have little time for leisurely pursuits, research or study . . ."

Dr. David Carrick, speaking at a public meeting in London, put it more succinctly. "None of us," he said, "is remotely happy."

13. To Promote the General Welfare

"Let's face it, most Americans today are simply fed up with government at all levels."

It was a candid admission for Richard Nixon, the most prominent symbol—and the most powerful caretaker—of that government. But the President, delivering his 1971 State of the Union message to the Congress, had touched on an important point. As he spoke of returning "power to the people," as he pledged that "once again in America we are placing our trust in people," he echoed the hopes of many frustrated and embittered citizens who had seen the government's promise "to promote the general welfare" subverted in a maze of legislation and bureaucracy that, in fact, had become increasingly harmful to both the *general* welfare and the welfare of the individual citizen.

Americans faced with proposals for massive new Federal health insurance programs can reflect on a lengthy history of costly government failure in other areas—welfare, public housing, mail delivery, farming—projects that have too frequently collapsed under the weight of faulty concepts, inept planning and inefficient administration.

Some examples are more prominent than others—more deeply etched in the public consciousness—because they have directly affected large segments of the populace and have won widespread notoriety. Most adult Americans, for example, can still recall the three-cent postage stamp and the "penny postcard." By 1971 the U.S. Postal Department had bogged down in a bureaucratic mire of more than 730,000 employees and annual expenditures of more than $8 billion—and Americans were paying eight cents to mail a letter (11 cents an ounce for airmail), and six cents for the "penny" postcard. Amazingly, as postal rates continued to soar, complaints about mail delivery became increasingly widespread.

In 1971, when Postmaster General Winton Blount announced plans to spend an additional billion dollars of the taxpayers' money to build new bulk-mail centers, independent businessman Thomas M. Murray, who had developed a highly successful private bulk-mail delivery service, stated that private enterprise could do the same job for one-fourth the cost and without using any taxpayer funds.

But the Post Office is not only costly, it is absurdly—and dangerously—inefficient. Award-winning reporter Clark Mollenhoff, a former member of President Nixon's White House staff, revealed in early 1971 that an administration decision to permit the processing of passports through the nation's post offices makes the passport system "a sitting duck for foreign agents and organized crime."

"Officials of the federal Passport Office report, after the first few months of the new system, errors by post office personnel have been occurring in about 15 to 18 percent of the passports issued," Mollenhoff reported.

The administration found that the Post Office Department had been lax in its selection of personnel and in maintaining its security system. Yet the findings should have come as no surprise. In 1969, Postmaster General Blount told a House committee that postal theft was widespread—within the post offices themselves. That year more than 1,100 postal employees were arrested for the theft of millions of dollars in merchandise and money. An attorney for the Justice Department, investigating postal thefts, reported that handling of registered mail was "incredible—very, very sloppy."

"Some government officials feel this lack of internal security in the post offices will make it easy for agents of organized crime and foreign governments to obtain passports," Mollenhoff warned. Yet the costly inefficiency of the postal system is only one of the more obvious examples of government failure.

Another failure of government has affected far fewer people—but those it has affected have felt the pain deeply. "When St. Louis' giant Pruitt-Igoe public housing complex was built in the 1950's," reported the *Dallas Morning News*, "it was hailed as a magnificent breakthrough for the housing of the poor; 33 multi-story apartment buildings, erected at a cost of $36 million to the taxpayer. Today it's called 'a high-rise hell.' Within three years after it opened a St. Louis newspaper described it as 'a paradise for thieves, thugs, and rapists and a nightmare for police' and the situation has deteriorated ever since."

An urban-affairs writer for the Associated Press has called the project "a shattered and torn symbol of all that's wrong and ruinous in the nation's public housing program."

And shattered and torn it is. "Stairwells and hallways became public toilets. Abandoned apartments became havens for dope pushers, hoods and sex criminals. Muggers preyed on the tenants. Gunfire echoed regularly from the upper floors of the half-deserted project," reported the *Morning News*.

By 1971, only 600 families lived in Pruitt-Igoe—a project designed to house more than 3,000 families. Repair estimates were placed at $39 million—three million dollars more than it cost to build the entire complex. Finally, the St. Louis Civil Alliance for Housing asked the Federal Government to tear the complex down. In a decade, the government's housing planners had succeeded only in providing a breeding ground for crime and wasting nearly $40 million of the taxpayers' money. An aide to George Romney, Secretary of the Department of Housing and Urban Development, referred to the project as a "lost ship" in the war on poverty. But when the planners received the request to dismantle the project, they made a counterproposal: spend another $22 million, they urged, to replace Pruitt-Igoe with more government-built housing units.

"If Washington decides to give Pruitt-Igoe a new ship—as past history suggests it will—taxpayers may be forgiven for wondering how long it will be before that's sunk, too," the *Morning News* said. "Though there may be a need for a new ship . . . it appears that there is an even more urgent need to do something about the wrecking crew that sank the first one."

But the wrecking crew—the cadre of housing planners who occupy the social drawing boards in Washington—is not to share the blame alone. The failure of the nation's public housing projects must be traced to the faulty concept that government bureaucracy can successfully solve problems. Michael Harrington, a disenchanted and frustrated liberal, complained about the failure of the government's housing programs in his widely read book *The Other America*. "Most public housing, even at its best, fails to solve the problem of the slum, and above all, the problem of slum psychology," Harrington wrote. "In some cases the gains appear minimal, for one must balance the physical improvement against the new forms of alienation and, at the extreme, of violence."

Harrington complained that under the government's housing and urban renewal programs—ostensibly designed to aid the poor —"it is the poor who are victimized." Urban renewal, he complained, displaces the poor to make way for dwellings the poor cannot afford. Thus the program sets off a migration within the cities, as slum families are forced to find new places to live. One St. Louis project—the Mill Creek urban renewal program—resulted in the displacement of a large number of Negro families, Harrington wrote. Of the uprooted families, half disappeared from the sight of city and Federal officials—probably forced to migrate to other cities. Only 14 percent ended up in other low-cost projects in St. Louis, he said.

Harrington's findings were echoed by Columbia Professor Martin Anderson, later to become a top White House aide, in his book *The Federal Bulldozer*. Anderson, too, found that the victims of urban renewal were the poor themselves. The urban renewal program, he concluded, "has actually made it more difficult for low-income and middle-income groups to obtain housing. It has done this by destroying much more of this kind of housing than it has created. Its net result has been to aggravate the housing shortage for those who have the most trouble finding suitable accommodations."

The Federal urban renewal program has extended into many thousands of American cities, displacing millions of Americans from their homes. "Many of the families that are required to move go into housing as bad as or worse than their original homes in other neighborhoods," Anderson wrote. "And they often pay higher rents at the new location."

The failing is not merely in the execution of the program. Like all government projects, urban renewal labors under an insurmountable handicap of politics and bureaucracy. The program should be repealed, Anderson urged. "No new projects should be authorized; the program should be phased out by completing, as soon as possible, all current projects. The federal urban renewal program conceived in 1949 had admirable goals. Unfortunately it has not achieved them in the past and cannot achieve them in the future. Only free enterprise can."

As the government has attempted to provide housing—and now seeks to provide medical care—it has also attempted to wipe out poverty. The results have been equally dismal.

One of the fronts on which the government undertook to increase the well-being of the indigent was the much-heralded "War on Poverty," launched by President Lyndon Johnson in a burst of optimism early in 1964. (It was actually a rekindled optimism, since Johnson's political mentor, the late President Franklin D. Roosevelt, had earlier launched his own unsuccessful government War on Poverty.)

Only two years after Johnson's administration resolved to launch a program that would provide jobs for the poor and wipe out poverty, the administration's leading spokesman in the U.S. Senate, Montana Senator Mike Mansfield, confessed that the government had apparently been "in too big a hurry." Job Corps centers had turned into centers for vandalism and Mansfield complained to the Senate, "It was not my intention to support the establishment of three reformatories in my state." Training provided by the Federal Job Corps was substandard and inadequate. In her book *Poverty Is Where the Money Is*, Shirley Scheibla, a highly regarded Washington correspondent, reported that the government's trainees were unable satisfactorily to fill the jobs they had been told they were being prepared for. Among her findings:

—Of 189 graduates of the Job Corps center in Charleston, West Virginia, only 70 had been able to find jobs as of the end of 1966.

—A corporate official reported that his company had paid for transportation of girl graduates to the firm's plant and helped the girls find housing, but learned that none were able to meet required proficiency standards, even after an additional 50-day on-the-job training period and a special 30-day training extension. Every one of the Job Corps graduates had to be dismissed—by a company that had a previous termination record of less than five percent.

—The manager of a photography shop reported that a "graduate of the center's photography course" had apparently had no photography training at all. The shop decided to train her at its own expense, and even bought her new clothes to wear on the job, but "she made no effort to learn." Finally she was fired.

—One research firm was using a Job Corps "draftsman" as a tracer. The firm reported it had been unable to find any of the Corps' graduate draftsmen who were capable of drafting.

—In 1966, when the Office of Economic Opportunity provided the Senate Labor and Welfare Committee with a list of companies that had supplied employment to graduates of the Job Corps' Breckenridge and Atterbury centers, Senator Everett Dirksen made a random check on four employers and found that the trainees had all been unsuited for the work and unwilling to learn—and all had lasted less than three weeks.

—A Congressional investigation in 1965 revealed that the Atterbury camp had more staff members (500) than trainees (300), and that the Breckenridge center had only slightly more trainees than staff, 358 to 350. Senator Strom Thurmond reported that the director of the Breckenridge camp had added his wife and the wives of 51 other staff members to the payroll.

—Packard Bell, which had won the contract for operating the Charleston center, on the basis of a $100,000 cost estimate, had spent nearly a quarter of a million dollars on the project by November, 1966.

—Costs for rehabilitating property for Job Corps centers in Poland Spring, Maine, came to $1.2 million—twice the original estimate. At Excelsior Springs, Missouri, the rehabilitation cost exceeded the estimates by $100,000—an overrun of 25 percent.

—Representative Thomas Pelly complained that the government spent nearly $2 million to send 13,000 Job Corps trainees home for the Christmas holidays in 1965, though servicemen on leave from Vietnam or military posts did not receive transportation money for travel in the U.S. Many servicemen, trying to get home for Christmas by using the airlines' stand-by, half-price tickets, were bumped from airplanes by Job Corps trainees with full-fare, government-paid tickets.

—Job Corps trainees could receive as much as $100 a month while in training (in addition to free transportation, housing, clothing, recreation, and medical and dental care). An Army private, on the other hand, received $94 a month.

—Representative Paul Fino complained that the Office of Economic Opportunity spent $370,000 to buy 30,000 brass-buttoned blazers for its 17,000 enrollees, at a time when the Army was suffering a uniform shortage.

—A Louis Harris survey found that 56 percent of Job Corps members had been working before entering the Corps for government training, but that only 54 percent were working after completing the government course. "Almost one in five feel they are worse off now than before they went into the Job Corps," the study revealed. In addition, 42 percent said they didn't get the training they had been promised, and 16 percent claimed they had not received any noticeable training at all. Only six percent of the Job Corps graduates kept their ensuing jobs for more than six months; the median job duration was less than two and one-half months.

Mark Sullivan, a member of the Board of Trustees of the OEO's United Planning Organization, in Washington, D.C., quit the War on Poverty in November, 1966, complaining that the organization "does little planning and conducts its operations inefficiently and at great administrative cost.

"As a consequence," he said, "funds designed to help the poor instead subsidize a vast and growing bureaucracy."

Shirley Scheibla found what others had found. For example, Rod Manis, a Stanford economist, told a Rampart College seminar, "Government is the greatest enemy of the poor. Its taxes, regulations, and expenditures are the primary obstacles the poor face in trying to better their lot. Americans have, for too long, been convinced that any problem can be solved with government bureaucracy and tax money. Perhaps the bitter reality of the poor's plight will force us to give up this dangerous illusion."

As examples, Manis pointed to the effect of government laws regulating trade union activity and minimum wage scales. "The government gives unions the power to exclude poor and minority workers from jobs," he said, pointing out that while white middle-class union members earn up to $20,000 a year, and strike for more, employers are prohibited from hiring non-union poor blacks who need the work.

Citing 1969 figures in *Newsweek* magazine, which revealed that only 5,000 of 130,000 youths in construction industry apprenticeship programs were black, Manis charged that government favoritism toward labor unions has created monopoly power through which unions have become "the primary bottleneck to the advancement of poor blacks in the cities." At the same time, minimum wage laws have sharply increased unemployment among the poorly trained poor. If an employer is required to pay an employee $1.60 an hour, for example, he cannot hire workers capable of producing only $1.00 worth of value in that time. A study reported by the *New York Times* in 1967 revealed that more than 100,000 poor farm workers in the South had lost their jobs because employers could not afford to keep them on at government-decreed minimum wage levels.

Manis reported similar findings by others:

—Gordon E. Brown, in his book *The Multi-Problem Dilemma*, found that welfare weakens incentives of recipients to find work by reducing welfare payments whenever a recipient earns money on his own; that it encourages the breakup of families by offering aid only if the father leaves the home; that social workers snoop into and control the lives of the poor, without providing much benefit in return.

—Martin Luther King, Jr., in his book *Where Do We Go From Here?*, claimed that American schools—established and run by state and local governments—"do not know how to teach."

—Paul Goodman, in his book *Compulsory Miseducation*, claimed that "in many underprivileged schools the IQ steadily falls the longer they go to school."

In fact, Manis' study indicates that the entire scope of government involvement in the lives of its citizens has produced a giant mural of failure. "Farm subsidies are supposed to help farmers," he says. "In fact, 85 percent goes to farms whose average sales exceed $10,000 while only 7 percent is spread thinly among those selling less than $5,000 a year."

The Federal Government has no better record in caring for the American Indian. Citing a 1966 report of the Senate Interior Committee and a 1969 study in the *Los Angeles Times*, Manis points out that the Bureau of Indian Affairs employs four bureaucrats for every 100 Indians—yet the Indian life expectancy is far less than that of white Americans, their average income is only one-third that of other Americans, only one-fourth are "employable," and 40 percent of that one-fourth are unemployed—after a century of government "care."

In the words of noted economist Milton Friedman, "I do not know of a single example of a predominantly collectivist or centrally planned society in which the ordinary citizen has achieved a major and substantial improvement in the condition of his everyday life or a real hope for the future of himself or his children."

Dr. Clarence B. Carson, Professor of History at Grove City (Pa.) College, came to similar conclusions in his book *The War on the Poor.*

"The war upon the poor will be ended when numerous interventions are ended," Carson concluded. ". . . Governments must be restricted to their proper sphere in order that the poor, as well as everyone else, may be freed to improve their own condition, if that is their desire . . .

"The hope of the poor lies with freedom. The politics of expansive government is not for the poor. Politics is the arena of influence peddlers, of batteries of lawyers, of five-percenters, of special tax exemptions for oil millionaires, of cost-plus contracts, of those who have the inside track, of demagogues who feather their nests at public expense, of the powers that be. The poor have neither the resources, the background and education, nor the time to spend on such quests. They cannot compete in this arena; at best, they will only get some of the crumbs that fall from the table . . ."

From the Postal Department to the Poverty Program and Urban Renewal, Uncle Sam has proven to be a wasteful spendthrift, unable to manage his own affairs efficiently and economically, and far less able to manage the affairs of others. The examples are seemingly endless:

—Early in 1971, syndicated columnists Rowland Evans and Robert Novak revealed that an OEO office in Los Angeles—the Los Angeles Neighborhood Legal Services Agency—was "a government-subsidized forum for revolutionary agitation." The office—designed to provide legal advice to the poor—was being used as a headquarters for a militant anti-draft organization. One of the group's members, a member of the radical Students for a Democratic Society [SDS], had allegedly attended Communist meetings in the U.S. and participated in Communist-sponsored trips to East Germany and Russia. Among his "clients" was a girl charged with contempt of court in a case involving the purchase of explosives by the even more radical Weathermen. The girl had been earning nearly $800 a month working for the Los Angeles municipal government—but taxpayers, who foot the bill for the OEO's activities, were saddled with her defense fees.

—In 1962, the government's General Accounting Office reported that a seven-acre field had been purchased by a nudist club and, because the acreage was taken out of grain production to make room for its other activities, the club received payments under the Agricultural Adjustment Act, that unique piece of legislation that pays farmers not to grow crops.

—Government accounting and record-keeping is so sloppy that when Congressman John Erlenborn tried to track down a reported $44,000 OEO expenditure for anti-tuberculosis work in DuPage County, Illinois, he found, after almost a year of search, that the money had actually gone into an educational experiment in another county.

—The government food stamp program, designed for the sole purpose of supplementing the diets of the poor and helping to prevent malnutrition, cost the American taxpayer $75 million in 1964. The next year the budget was $100 million. Then $200 million. It was $225 million in 1967; $315 million in 1968; $340 million in 1969; $610 million in 1970. By 1971, the food stamp budget was $1.7 billion—an increase of 2,200 percent in eight years. During a 1970 General Motors strike, the government alloted $14 million worth of food stamps not to the unemployed poor, but to workers who had voluntarily walked off well-paying jobs in an attempt to make them better-paying jobs.

—Senator Walter F. Mondale revealed in 1971 that the Department of Health, Education and Welfare had used funds from a $75 million emergency school-desegregation program to buy a $15,000 mobile zoo and $300,000 in school television equipment—"having nothing whatsoever to do with the problems of desegregation."

—Columnist Victor Riesel revealed in early 1971 that scores of Federal agents, dispatched by the General Accounting Office, were searching for documentation for expenditures of $144 million in poverty funds, the bulk of which "is simply unaccounted for, simply unquestioned by the Office of Economic Opportunity auditors over the years . . . There are just no records. There just are no receipts. There just is no justification for trips, expenditures and other 'items.' " According to Riesel, "the figure is expected to run up to $200 million in mishandled funds . . ."

—A report on the effectiveness of 15 Department of Health, Education and Welfare programs, prepared by a team of college students and community workers, found that a majority of children participating in the migrant-education program were not migrant children; that Head Start classes were packed with ineligible children; that education funds that were to be allocated to schools based on the number of disadvantaged pupils enrolled in the school were, in fact, being distributed without regard to the number of disadvantaged children; that program directors were frequently ignoring Congressional guidelines.

—Inflationary government economic policies have caused factory workers to lose ground in terms of actual take-home income, despite steadily "increasing" wages. Department of Labor statistics released in 1971 revealed that while average weekly wages rose approximately from $130 to $134 between 1969 and 1970, in terms of 1957–59 dollars, "actual" income dropped from slightly over $100 to approximately $98.

—The costly paper shuffling of government bureaucracy descends to such ludicrous depths that Congressman H.R. Gross recently chided the Office of Economic Opportunity for an interdepartmental memorandum that read: "It has come to my attention that your office is 16 letters overdue in responding to the Director's correspondence. Effective immediately all personnel in the Office of Health Affairs are denied permission for any travel regarding official OEO business until Health Affairs' overdue mail is brought down to 15 letters or under." (It makes one wonder just how important "official" OEO travel actually is, if it can be so matter-of-factly suspended for tardiness in answering memos; in fact, it makes one wonder how important the memos themselves are, if it takes an accumulation of 16 unanswered letters to prompt official concern.)

These are no isolated examples, collected over a period of years.

They are but a few of the illustrations of government ineptitude that were reported in the public press during the first three months of 1971. Every day, Americans are exposed to additional examples of government's inability to cope with the duties we have surrendered to it.

Nor is the failure of government restricted to the national level. New York City residents, after successive reports that (a) a public works project for the city would cost up to $150 million more than was budgeted, due to "errors," and (b) the city's manpower program had disintegrated into a "fragmented, disjointed, overlapping conglomerate," learned that (c) the city's "Human Resources Administration" had been bedding welfare families in the posh Waldorf Astoria Hotel at a cost of more than $76 a day: total cost, $12,000 a year to provide more than 1,000 welfare recipients with New York's most exclusive living quarters.

Government, created by the people, has become master instead of servant, at great cost to the public in terms both of money and freedom.

Willard Edwards of the *Chicago Tribune* recently reported the plight of an elderly immigrant, 70-year-old Paul Tobeler. "He worked hard all his life, accumulated savings, and invested them in two apartment buildings near the University of Southern California," wrote Edwards. Four student tenants suddenly refused to pay their rent, claiming the building was not in sufficient repair. Tobeler gave them a choice: if they didn't want to pay the back rent they could simply find new apartments. The government (the OEO's Western Center on Law and Poverty—created to help the poor with legal problems) rounded up twenty additional tenants, instigated a rent strike, and filed a class action lawsuit against Tobeler, overwhelming him with a "barrage of legal documents" that threatened him with contempt if he refused to allow the students to use his property.

"With courts congested," Edwards wrote, "the lawsuit would not be settled for years. During that time, Tobeler . . . would have to continue making mortgage payments, pay taxes and utilities, provide managers and services to run the premises. Bankruptcy and loss of his property were inevitable."

Tobeler's attorneys argue that he is being used as a "guinea pig in litigation brought by and financed by the OEO for the apparent purpose of effectuating social change in the economic and legal structure of this country . . ." Meanwhile, the taxpayers pay for the lawsuit filed by Tobeler's tenants.

Tobeler is not the only victim of an apparently omnipresent government. Senator Sam Ervin complained early in 1971 that many Americans are beginning to protest government snooping into their private affairs. Ervin complained that the U.S. Census Bureau had been harassing newly retired persons with questions about missing teeth, artificial dentures, number of telephone calls made by children to their parents, and extent of personal happiness or unhappiness. The pensioners are harassed by mail and telephone until they answer, Ervin charged.

Not only does the public suffer at the hands of its inefficient and domineering government, it pays a high price for the privilege. The Tax Foundation, Inc., a highly respected private research organization, reported that the average American taxpayer would work two hours and 37 minutes of every eight-hour workday during 1971 just to pay the cost of maintaining his governments. At that rate, the worker earning $10,000 a year would pay more than $13 for taxes out of every $40 earned: $8.70 earmarked for the federal government and $4.35 for state and local governments. The amount of the daily wage taken for taxes, the foundation said, would be nearly two and one-half times the amount spent for food and tobacco; more than two and one-half times the amount spent for housing; more than four times the amount spent for transportation; more than six times the amount spent for clothing; *approximately seven times the amount spent for medical care;* more than eight times the amount spent for personal recreation.

What's more, the situation is probably going to get worse. Robert R.G.M. Statham, a tax expert with the U.S. Chamber of Commerce, has estimated that the average American family's income will rise by about 60 percent in the next decade—but that federal, state and local taxes will increase by *100* percent.

Implicit in the call for national health insurance is the assumption that government "can do it better." Yet history proves the opposite. Government's record is one of wastefulness and inefficiency.

Perhaps it is wrong to expect more. While Americans have long criticized the increasing centralization of national power, they have been too infrequently aware of a corresponding decentralization—

a diffusion of the Federal power into hundreds of boards, bureaus and agencies that work anonymously to produce the regulations, directives and decrees by which government actually governs. Under such a system, businessmen, farmers and physicians too frequently find their training subordinated to the second-guessing expertise of clerks conducting their daily duties in compliance with rigid departmental guidelines.

Of course, not all bureaucrats are incompetent; most who reach levels of discretionary authority may be as capable as their counterparts in the private sector of life. But the bureaucracy itself predominates, and talent and skill are too often buried under volumes of paperwork and detailed procedures. In such a system it is understandable that mountains of memos could pass unanswered from department to department; that millions of dollars could be spent without the government really knowing how—or to whom —the funds were disbursed; that offices built to combat poverty could be used to defend violent militancy.

Those who criticize isolated instances of government failure as they occur—and marvel at the frequency of such occurences—fail to recognize that the fault is in the system itself; that wastefulness, incompetence and inefficiency are an integral part of any attempt by a massive, depersonalized bureaucracy to provide for distinctly human individuals in cities and towns many hundred of miles from the seats of power.

In his book *The Great Farm Problem*, William Peterson wrote: "A generation of 'farm policy' adds up to hopeless tinkering, fantastic losses, planned chaos, a lost war against Nature's laws . . . The irony is that the farmer to be saved wasn't; since the New Deal, one of every three farmers has quit."

Similar results can be expected in other areas as well. Today loud voices call for massive government intervention into the highly technical realm of providing medical care for human beings. Government's record in other fields should cause advocates of national health insurance to consider carefully the possible dangers of such a course.

14. The Medicare Experience

Americans who wish a preview of the effect national health insurance is likely to have on medical care in this country need not look solely to the dismal record of similar health programs in European nations. America, too, has had its experience with government medicine. In 1965, after more than half a century of study and debate, the United States enacted its first major nationwide program of government-financed health care. Within less than five years that program—Medicare—had pushed up health care costs, endangered the financial stability of non-profit hospitals, repeatedly boosted membership fees paid by the nation's aged (who had been forced to rely on the program for their medical care) and had run up staggering bills, far above initial estimates.

Medicare is already an acknowledged failure—almost as much so as its legislative twin, the Medicaid program for the indigent, which has driven administering state governments to the brink of economic collapse. So poorly have the programs fared that in early 1970, Robert Finch, then Secretary of Health, Education, and Welfare, was forced to admit:

"The Federal government is spending over $10 billion this year to buy health care for the aged and the poor under the Medicare and Medicaid programs. This is double what was estimated when these programs were enacted in 1965, just five years ago. In another five years, given the present trend, the cost will be at least $20 billion.

"We are not getting our money's worth. The aged and the poor are not getting all of the care they need."

The failure of the program should have come as no surprise to its sponsors. The failings—overutilization, mismanagement, sky-rocketing costs—are integral parts of the system. They have been present in government health programs for centuries. One need not go back to the failure of the Devon experiment in 1769 (see Appendix I) to find evidence of the problems that inevitably accompany government medicine; the advocates of national health insurance, and the advocates of Medicare before them, can find ample illustration in the experience of the Veterans Administration program in this country.

In a 1971 report entitled "Our VA Hospitals Are in Trouble," *Reader's Digest* concluded that "the system is beset by critical malfunctions that result in misspent funds and misdirected treatment." The report, based on a five-month survey, included three revealing case histories:

—In Los Angeles, a 50-year-old World War II veteran suffering from pneumonia died of suffocation when the Veterans Administration hospital, hard pressed to find enough nurses for routine duty, could not provide the special nursing care needed to suction accumulating mucus from a breathing tube inserted in the patient's throat.

—In Philadelphia, equipment breakdowns and shortages of hospital technicians and pathologists resulted in a VA patient remaining in bed for a month for abdominal surgery that would have required less than half the time at a private hospital.

—Because VA regulations do not permit "outpatient" treatment for such illnesses, a young Korean War veteran suffering a mild asthma attack had to be admitted as a patient in order to receive medical care. He stayed in the hospital for three days at a time when the hospital was nearly filled to capacity.

The stories are not untypical. *Reader's Digest* reports that these three cases are only part of a file of hundreds of similar stories that have led to widespread criticism of the VA hospital system. Among the report's major points:

—Doctors and nurses, reporting on extensive private studies and carrying affidavits of colleagues, have complained to Congress that veterans are receiving "woefully inadequate" medical care in old, understaffed and ill-equipped hospitals.

—Senator Alan Cranston, chairman of a Senate investigation into the conduct of VA hospitals, has reported that "conditions in many veterans hospitals are deplorable."

—The VA's Department of Medicine and Surgery complains that budget policies have "imposed serious fiscal constraints on our abilities to employ adequate personnel and provide necessary facilities."

—Dr. Baldwin Lamson, director of hospitals and clinics at UCLA, has testified that the nursing staff at the VA hospital in Los Angeles is "approximately one half" of the number considered "essential."

—Dr. Stanley J. Dudrick, chief of surgery at the VA hospital in Philadelphia, complains that the hospital has "insufficient equipment, insufficient personnel and grossly inadequate support" in the radiology, pathology and clinical laboratory areas.

—Dr. Thomas A. Gonda, Associate Dean of the Stanford University Medical School, has called radiology equipment at the VA hospital in Palo Alto "obsolete in the worst sense of the word, broken down in every true sense."

—Salary restrictions hinder VA hospitals in recruiting personnel, often resulting in a lapse of months before staff vacancies can be filled, whereas community hospitals can fill similar vacancies in "a matter of days."

—During the first ten months of 1970, the VA hospital in West Roxbury, Massachusetts, reported a 190 percent turnover of nurses' aides in one major department.

—An out-of-date blood analyzer at one VA hospital was out of order for 10 percent of the time during one six-month period in 1970, causing testing delays that resulted in patients needlessly occupying beds "at a financial loss to the taxpayer and themselves."

—Delays in pre-surgical tests, caused by a shortage of technicians, resulted in a 15 percent increase in the length of hospital stays in the new VA hospital in Miami, Florida.

—X-ray series that technicians claim should be completed in a single day often take from three to ten days in VA hospitals because of faulty equipment and inadequate personnel. (*Reader's Digest* quotes a chief of medicine at one VA hsopital as complaining that the delay would not be tolerated in any private hospital in his community.)

—Doctors and nurses at every major VA hospital studied by the magazine told reporter Kenneth Tomlinson that as many as one-fourth of the patients in their hospitals needn't be there: alcoholics, the elderly, and veterans with minor ailments. (One of every eight patients in VA hospitals is an alcoholic.)

—Ambitious administrators often do everything they can to keep beds *full* (a practice *Reader's Digest* describes as "bureaucratic gamesmanship") because the system provides hospital financing on the basis of bed occupancy.

—More than half of the system's 166 hospitals are more than 30 years old.

—Thirty-six hospitals, many of them in hot southern climates, have no air conditioning.

Government medical programs—like all government programs —are based on politics. VA hospitals, for example, have been built in:

—Marlin, Texas (population 6,000)—because the late Senator Tom Connally wanted a VA hospital in his hometown, even though Marlin is within 40 minutes of an 800-bed hospital in Temple and a 1,000-bed hospital in Waco;

—Miles City, Montana (population: 9,000—because the late Senator James Murray wanted it there;

—Dublin, Georgia (population 10,000)—because Rep. Carl Vinson, then chairman of the House Armed Services Committee, wanted it there.

Donald E. Johnson, administrator of the VA, tries to blame the system's failings on "the national medical care crisis." But the facts point the finger of guilt at the system itself. For example, the increased costs indicated by the extended hospital stays uncovered in the *Reader's Digest* study are clearly substantiated by other reports as well. In 1970, the New Orleans Council of Medical Staffs, headed by Dr. Jose Garcia Oller, a highly regarded neurosurgeon, conducted a comparative study of hospitalization costs at that city's hospitals (see Chapter 10). The report concluded that although the per diem charge for hospital care was considerably lower in the government hospitals, the *duration* of stay was much longer, resulting in significantly higher costs for treatment in either of the government hospitals (one VA hospital and one Public Health Service hospital).

The figures:

Hospital	Per Diem		Average Stay		Cost per stay
Ochsner	$67.0	×	9.61 days	=	$644
Touro	78.1	×	8.20	=	640
Hotel Dieu	71.2	×	7.74	=	551
Flint	49.6	×	10.40	=	516
Baptist	60.9	×	7.90	=	·481
Mercy	68.0	×	6.86	=	466
Sara Mayo	64.2	×	6.10	=	392

****

Charity	45.3	×	14.10	=	639

****

USVAH	49.6	×	22.00	=	1,091
USPHS	52.0	×	17.70	=	920

In summary, even though the per diem rate in the government hospitals was lower ($50.80 on the average, compared with $63), the longer average hospital stay (19.85 days, compared with 8.86 days), meant that patients in government hospitals, or the taxpayers who foot the bills, paid considerably more for the average period of hospitalization ($1,008, compared with an average of only $541 in the non-government hospitals). A patient who received his hospital treatment under government medicine spent an additional 11 days in the hospital, often at considerable cost in lost work time, as well as incurring an additional dollar cost of $467.

(These figures compare government hospitals with non-government hospitals. A comparison between "free" hospitals and non-"free" hospitals would drop Charity, which has the longest average stay and third-highest average cost among non-government hospitals, from the first list and add it to the second, thus increasing the disparity.)

The New Orleans study also revealed that the lengthy hospital stays caused by the inadequate equipment, personnel shortages and other shortcomings uncovered in the *Reader's Digest* report—as well as the patient's own tendency to linger when his care is free—have put a heavy strain on the hospitals themselves. For example, the New Orleans VA hospital had an occupancy rate of 84.5 percent at the time of the study. If the average stay had been reduced from the 22-day figure to 9.6 days (the same as at Ochsner Hospital), occupancy would have dropped to 36.9 percent, freeing many beds. If the average stay were 8.2 days (the same as at Touro), the occupancy rate would have dropped still further, to 31.5 percent, and if the average stay were 6.1 days, the same as at Sara Mayo Hospital, the occupancy rate would have been only 23.4 percent. Similar findings were reported for the U.S. Public Health Service hospital, which would have reduced occupancy rates from the actual 77 percent to 41.8, 36.1 and 26.5 percent, respectively.

A study reported by Dr. Kenneth Ray, of Detroit, in 1969, produced similar findings. "In the past 20 years," Dr. Ray wrote, "the medical profession has been subjected to an increasing amount of criticism, primarily from two sources . . . the federal government and organized labor . . . Ironically, neither the federal government nor organized labor has . . . shown much concern for efficiency in their own operations."

In a comparative study of 37 Detroit-area hospitals, Dr. Ray found the two most expensive to be the Veterans Administration hospital and the Metropolitan Hospital, a facility established by Detroit labor leaders "to demonstrate to organized medicine how medical care could be delivered at a cut rate."

A prime feature of government health programs is the "closed" staff hospital, in which use of facilities is limited to salaried physicians, working directly for the hospital, in contrast to the more common "open" staff hospitals, including most community hospitals, which allow local physicians to treat patients in their facilities. The limited or "closed" staff is also a key feature of many prepayment group medical clinics, and has been widely advocated by sponsors of government health plans as a means of increasing efficiency and reducing costs. Using figures reported by the hospitals themselves to the American Hospital Association, Ray drew revealing comparisons between Detroit's "open" and "closed" hospitals:

"When all open staff hospitals are compared to closed staff hospitals, with salaried physicians, a striking disparity appears. The average cost per admission at closed staff hospitals is $1,197, while the average of all open staff hospitals is under $550. This represents a difference of over 100 percent . . .

"The two prime critics of the present method of delivering medical care have an interest in this comparison. The federal government owns and operates the VA Hospital in Allen Park. Their cost of $3,350 per admission (despite the lowest ratio of employees per patient) is over three times the cost of the highest open staff hospital. Moreover, they do not have a coronary care unit. The Metropolitan Hospital is a facility of the Community Hospital Association which was established by Walter Reuther and his associates . . . At $1,309 per admission, their cost is almost twice the highest open staff hospital cost, and earns them second place on the list. They also do not have a coronary care unit. The fact that Metropolitan Hospital has 5.58 employees per patient suggests they may also have labor troubles." (Most hospitals in the survey reported a range of 2.5 to 3 employees per patient.)

"Closed staff hospitals, where physicians are on a salary, have a significantly higher cost than open staff community hospitals," Dr. Ray concluded. "This discrepancy prevails in spite of the facilities offered or the role of the hospital in the community.

"Among the self-appointed experts in Medical care at the national level," he wrote, "there is a growing support for group practice. The extremists of this element advocate a program in which the physician is a salaried employee of the hospital. The proponents of these plans claim that this would improve the delivery of medical care and imply that this would also reduce medical costs . . . On the contrary, there is a clear indication that the most certain way to double hospital costs would be to put the attending staff on a salary. As regards the VA hospital, it appears that these patients could receive their care in a good community hospital, the patient could be paid his salary during his hospitalization, and the government would still save $1,000 per patient admission. The saving at the one hospital in Allen Park after meeting all of these qualifications would be $6,095,000 per year."

VA hospitals and Public Health Service facilities are prime examples of the inefficiency and high cost that flow from government health programs. But there are other problems as well, and they are not limited to such massive programs.

Skyrocketing costs and political control nearly closed Chicago's huge government-run Cook County Hospital in mid-1970, after bitter disputes between the hospital's medical personnel and political overseers. The long battle led to a mass resignation by most of the hospital's 450 interns and residents and 70 attending physicians, caused the popular hospital superintendent to quit in anger, and threatened to leave more than 1,700 indigent patients without hospital care. What is more, warned *Medical World News*, the Cook County Board of Commissioners "may be only the first of many supervisory panels to face this dilemma. Cook County Hospital has its counterparts—more or less—in major metropolitan areas around the country."

The Cook County Hospital is huge—22 buildings, 6,000 employees, more than 2,200 beds—"a graying, ramshackle plant with corridors scarred by peeling paint and permeated by what can only be described as an odor of poverty." Frank Blatchford III, a reporter for the *Chicago Tribune,* summed up the problem in an article in *Private Practice.*

"Over the years," Blatchford wrote, "the hospital had become as much a tool in the hands of politicians as it was a facility designed to care for the poor. Property owners paid their taxes, the county politicians ran the hospital, and nobody got very upset if the politicians used the nonmedical hospital jobs as building blocks for their patronage empire, or if the patients were packed into the wards like sardines."

Robert J. Freeark became superintendent of the hospital in September, 1968, the appointee of reform-minded Richard Ogilvie (later elected Governor of Illinois). Freeark knew the mess he faced and joined Ogilivie's battle to rid the hospital of political control. "All the time I was an intern and on the staff of the hospital, after every election there would be a whole new turnover of employees," he said. "The major objection I have to the patronage system is the attitude it fosters in the employees. Their loyalty is to the guy who got them the job, not to the hospital. They figure it's all right to goof off and steal because they think, 'I've got to make this job pay off now, because after the next election I may not hold it anymore.' "

But Freeark was fighting a tough battle. If he wanted to hire anyone he had to clear the appointment with the politicians. "All the hiring was handled downtown by the patronage office," he said. Sometimes the order was just the opposite. "My personnel director would tell me, 'We've got orders from the patronage office to fire four employees. They say these are patronage jobs they want to fill with their people.' "

Freeark also found himself a victim of the inevitable bureaucracy that dominates all government-financed programs and that would be a certain aspect of any national health program. He was faced with trying to operate his hospital efficiently under a budget drawn up by laymen who (a) were unfamiliar with the problems of hospital management, and (b) had other concerns uppermost in their minds. "The budget would call for 50 custodial workers," Freeark complained. "We could probably have done the job with 10 persons if we had paid them a little more, but it was to the advantage of the politicians to have 50 patronage jobs. Those 50 job holders were 50 potential precinct captains.

"That's how they really controlled things. We asked for a reclassification of 400 employees at the time of the 1970 budgets and were granted four. The concept that a county job classification agency that serves the courts and the forest preserve can also serve the hospital is an example of the board's outdated employment practices. Such a board can't possibly serve a hospital that it knows practically nothing about."

Freeark said patronage and budgeting problems reflected only part of the political mismanagement of the hospital. "In addition to the patronage and the inflexible budget, there's the whole business of purchasing and letting of contracts. It was amazing who was bidding on county jobs. The top architects and suppliers didn't want anything to do with them."

Freeark tells of the time the hospital kitchen ran out of canned tomatoes because the supplier couldn't meet the time schedule specified in the county's contract. Instead of assessing a penalty for the contract violation, the county purchasing agent simply assigned the job to the next-highest bidder. He explained that if the county penalized suppliers for failing to meet their contracts, "We wouldn't have any suppliers."

"Obviously, few firms were willing to do business with the county," Freeark learned.

Freeark and Ogilvie ran into stiff resistance in their efforts to operate the hospital professionally. "Let's not have any doubts about this," said George Dunne, chairman of the county commissioners. "We, and not a bunch of doctors, are running Cook County Hospital."

Frustrated, and gambling that his move would unite the various elements of the hospital into a firm stand, Freeark resigned on May 15, 1970. By June 5, a survey by *Medical World News* revealed that six of 11 surgical department heads had resigned, along with 23 of 31 surgical residents, and all residents in urology and otolaryngology. Many of the remaining staff physicians and residents indicated that they planned to quit, too. Pressed by a medical staff in revolt and spiraling costs—the operating budget had soared from $28.5 million in 1965 to more than $60 million for fiscal 1971—the Illinois legislature took control of the hospital's budget, personnel, and purchasing from the county politicians and granted the powers to an independent governing commission.

Blatchford summed up the Cook County lesson:

"Although tight-fisted control of hospitals by big-city political machines is almost surely a thing of the past, politicians and bureaucrats of all types will almost equally as surely be advancing plans for more and more government control of hospitals. When they do, we would be wise not to forget the experience at County."

The Cook County experience and the dismal record of the VA hospitals offer a clear warning to those who would substitute government health programs for the current medical system based predominantly on private enterprise. But the clearest lesson of all is offered by the nation's unhappy experience with Medicare and Medicaid.

Medicaid, for example, is a Federal program for providing health care for "the needy." Administration of the program is left to the individual states, which pay part of the cost on a matched-fund basis. The results have been nearly disastrous. In California, for example, the number of "needy" who have applied for—and received—admission to Medi-Cal (the state's Medicaid program) had topped 2.4 million people by early 1971—12 percent of the state's population. "Medi-Cal's costs have doubled in four years and are still climbing," the *San Francisco Examiner* cried. "The system could bankrupt the state . . ." (see Chapter 10).

Medi-Cal services are being abused, complained the *Examiner*, "simply because they are free." The abuse is clearly evident; the warnings that government-subsidized health programs produce widespread overutilization were clearly borne out by Medi-Cal's experience. In fiscal 1969-70, there were 141 claims filed for every 100 persons enrolled in the program! By June, 1969, a little more than three years after the plan was put into operation, California Blue Shield and Blue Cross, fiscal intermediaries for the program, had already processed more than 66 million Medi-Cal claims.

Blue Shield is responsible for processing claims for professional services; all claims for hospital and nursing home services are handled by Blue Cross. So many Californians have flocked to doctors' offices that in the first month of the plan's operation Blue Shield processed more than 74,000 claims a day—10 times its ordinary workload. By November, 1969, Blue Shield was using high-speed computers to process an average of 100,000 claims a day.

In 1967, the first full year of Medi-Cal, there were slightly more than one million Californians on the program's rolls. By 1970, there were nearly two and one-half million. Costs soared: in 1967 the program cost the state $600 million; by 1970, Medi-Cal was draining the state at the rate of $1.2 billion a year. The result was a rapid increase in individual medical costs. The *San Francisco Examiner* complained that support of the Medi-Cal program had driven the average Californian's health-care expenses up to a burdensome $517 a year by 1970, compared to only $312 per person for the rest of the nation. "It [Medi-Cal] has become a monster devouring the state's dollar resources," the newspaper warned. "Currently it is consuming an amount equal to the total sum raised by the state income tax."

Medi-Cal allows the poor to get a wider range of health care for free than the average working man can afford to pay for. For example, under Medi-Cal the State and Federal governments— meaning, of course, the taxpayers—pick up the cost of nursing home care, dental care, home health care, occupational therapy, optometrics, chiropractic care, special duty nursing, psychological care, drugs, hearing aids, physical therapy—even speech therapy— on a 100 percent-payment basis. No limits are placed on the length of hospital stay or physician fees, etc., although private health insurance companies limit the extent to which those services are covered for the working man who arranges for his own health care protection. Ironically, the *Examiner* points out, "The working man's taxes, which support Medi-Cal, are one reason he can't afford more health care."

California's experience with Medicaid is not unique. In early 1970, the Texas Public Welfare Commission announced that it was cutting state Medicaid benefits by some 20 percent in order to stave off an estimated $42 million deficit during the following 17 months. The cutback was averted by a last-minute decision of the Texas legislature to transfer $13.5 million—which had been appropriated for development of two new medical schools—to undergird the shaky Medicaid programs.

Other states, as well, began to feel the pinch.

—In Massachusetts and New Hampshire, state legislatures set new fee schedules that would permit the states arbitrarily to withhold payment of part of a physician's fees to keep the program from going bankrupt.

—New York State cut back sharply on the number of benefits offered and the number of people covered.

—Virginia discontinued offering dental benefits only a few months after the program was started.

—Iowa dropped its "medically indigent" from Medicaid rolls, covering only the state's welfare recipients.

—Louisiana cut back on the number of hospital days allowed, and stopped providing eyeglasses free under the program.

—Wisconsin tightened eligibility conditions.

—Washington placed a limit on the number of home visits by a physician that would be covered by the state's Medicaid program.

Medicaid rapidly became an acknowledged failure, from coast to coast. The Health Policy Advisory Center, in a 1970 report, summed it up: "Medicaid began in 1966 . . . Medicaid began to die two years . . . later."

The Medicaid program staggered New York just as its sister program had staggered California under the name of Medi-Cal.

The report stated that New York City, "which embraced Medicaid like a long lost brother, fell the hardest. . . . By the depth of its fall, it reveals most clearly what happened in other cities as well." The report quoted a veteran hospital physician as saying: "Medicaid set health care in New York City back thirty years. Now we're just picking up the pieces."

The Medicaid program in New York suffered from the plan's skyrocketing costs. In 1968 and 1969, the state legislature cut the program severely, removing more than 1.2 million New York City residents from the eligibility rolls. "Despite the fears of liberals," said the Health Policy Advisory Center report, "no one rioted. It was not that the poor were uninterested in medical care. They were just not impressed by Medicaid."

Medicaid, in fact, had not been impressive. Medical services that had once been offered free were now costly; the neighborhood health centers that the city had promised to build with Medicaid income remained a promise and nothing more (as had most of the community health centers promised under Britain's form of government medicine); no new services were offered; the quality of care remained essentially unchanged, and the costs soared. "The residue of Medicaid . . . is the wreckage of the city's forty-year-old public health and hospital system," the report charged. "The city has less to offer, to fewer people and at greater cost, than at any other time since the depression."

By mid-1970, the program had become such an embarrassment to advocates of government health systems that few people could be found to defend it. Despite the Federal Government's great hope for the program, state governments joined slowly and reluctantly. Even though Washington was to reimburse 50 percent of Medicaid costs to even the wealthiest states, and as much as 83 percent to states with lower per capita incomes, only seven states had established programs in January, 1966, when Medicaid went into effect. A year later, 24 states—nearly half of all—still had not joined the plan. As late as 1969, nine states still refused to get involved in the costly mess that Medicaid had rapidly become. (Finally, the Federal Government blackmailed most of the remainder into the program: Washington decreed that any state that had not submitted an acceptable Medicaid plan by January 1, 1970, would automatically lose all Federal funds for medical aid to dependent children, the blind and the disabled. By the end of December, 1969, seven of the remaining states gave up their resistance and adopted Medicaid programs. Only Alaska and Arizona refused to become a part of the growing Medicaid entanglement.)

The reluctance of state governments to join the program is understandable. The costs of Medicaid have been far higher than even its bitterest opponents had predicted. Expenditures for Medicaid had quadrupled from $1.3 billion in 1967 to $5.5 billion by January, 1970.

In January, 1971, the Federal Government reported that two

government programs—aid to families with dependent children and Medicaid—had accounted for more than 70 percent of the increase in welfare costs during 1970. These, of course, are measurable costs, reported in Federal health expenditure statistics, and obvious to any investigator. There are, however, other costs—less discernible but no less painful to the ultimate victim: the average citizen. For example, a prominent market research firm reported in 1970 that many drug stores have increased prescription drug prices for all their customers in order to make up for the cost of handling Medicaid claims and paperwork. (See Chapter 10.)

Medicaid, in short, has become a costly flop. According to Princeton Professor Herman Somers, "It's a prime example of a program ill-conceived and badly executed." But advocates of government health programs are not easily deterred. Though they concede the failure of Medicaid, they do not concede the failure of the concept that bred it. It is simply a program that did not go far enough, they say.

Medicaid is an amalgamation of programs within a program. Each state has its own rules for eligibility (if the entire nation adopted the New York rules, for example, it is estimated that nearly half the population would qualify as medically needy); its own schedule of benefits; its own intermediary systems. It is this failure to concentrate the planning into a single omnipotent (and presumably omniscient) agency that is blamed for the Medicaid fiasco by those who remain unshaken in their faith in government's ability to plan and provide health services. They also blame the fact that the program was limited. For example, Barbara and John Ehrenreich, vocal advocates of government medical systems, complain that Congress amended the Medicaid law to put a ceiling on the family incomes that would qualify for assistance. Even with the limitations, however, states were allowed to provide Medicaid coverage to persons with incomes a full one-third higher than state welfare cutoffs. Presumably the program would have worked better if it had been unlimited—if any person, regardless of his income or ability to pay, had been permitted to demand that the government pay his medical bills.

Such an assertion, of course, is ridiculous. The Medi-Cal rolls kept growing, and the costs kept climbing. New York City's Medicaid costs climbed so rapidly that the State legislature cut the program sharply, even though there *were* Congressional limits on eligibility. If the program had been open-ended, the costs would have been incalculable.

Medicaid's failure, according to those who want still more government medicine, is also due in part to the system within which it was forced to operate—meaning, of course, a system of freedom.

The Health Policy Advisory Center's report revealed that the advent of Medicaid caused some of New York City's poor to leave government hospitals for private care, but (a) *not enough* left to allow the city to close its municipal hospitals, as had been hoped, and (b) *too many* left to keep the municipal hospitals full. It costs nearly as much to maintain an empty bed as it does a full one, so the city government suffered a severe financial blow. The lesson is clear enough, yet it is one that social planners refuse to see: in a free society, men cannot be expected to move about exactly as their movements had been planned on a government drawing board. It is this failure to understand the nature of a free human being that has consistently thrown a monkey wrench into the Utopian plans of those who would reshape our free enterprise systems.

The arguments can be tested: if Medicaid's failure was due to insufficient control and diffused planning, then the remedying of those faults would presumably create a workable program of Federal health care subsidization. By those standards, the Medicare program should have become a booming success. On the contrary it, too, has failed.

Medicare, the 1965 law that provides Federally-paid health care for the aged, is a limited program of national health insurance. The rules are all made in Washington. Though liberals speak freely of the failures of Medicaid, they are not so outspoken about the equally obvious failure of Medicare. The Medicare program offers the presumably "ideal" situation that is so lacking in Medicaid—a single central program. To speak of Medicare's failure is to call into serious question the entire concept of national health programs. Yet the program *has* failed.

In a bulky 323-page report issued in February, 1970, the Senate Finance Committee charged that *both* Medicare and Medicaid were "in serious financial trouble" and that both were having a seriously adverse effect on the health care costs paid by the general public. That same month, John C. Venaman, Undersecretary of the Department of Health, Education and Welfare, admitted to the Senate that the Medicare program, if it continues on its present course, will have a $217 billion deficit by 1995. Mel Schechter, a Washington health affairs expert, writing in *The New Republic*, predicted the deficit would be even worse—$236 billion for hospital-related benefits alone. Experience with the program "has demonstrated that radical change in medical practice can bring complications that had not been anticipated, particularly skyrocketing costs far beyond original estimates," warned the *New York Times*.

Medicare has created three major health care problems: serious financial difficulties for hospitals, decreased quality of care for the aged, and soaring costs for everybody.

Administrators of the nation's private hospitals have warned repeatedly that inadequate compensation under the Medicare program is seriously jeopardizing not only the quality of hospital care, but also efficiency, technological progress, medical education, and expansion. "For physicians who use hospital facilities, the implications are clear," wrote Harry C. Knickerbocker, Jr., author of a 1969 report. "If the administrator's claims are valid, the quality of health care doctors can administer will be severely limited."

The problem stems from the fact that Medicare reimburses hospitals only for costs, not for their normal charges for service. T.H. Morrison, administrator of Valley Baptist Hospital, in Harlingen, Texas, wrote to the Social Security Administration in 1969, asking that the hospital be dropped from the list of facilities providing care to Medicare beneficiaries. "The cost finding systems, formulas, guidelines and conditions of participation . . . penalize efficiency, quality patient care, proven management capabilities and integrity," Morrison wrote, "whereas incompetency, inefficiency, excessive and unjustified costs are compensated, rewarded and even glorified . . ."

Morrison, who has spent nearly 40 years in hospital administration, complained that, "To continue in the existing program . . . and remain financially responsible, efficient, adequately equipped and staffed, would be wholly impossible." If the hospital opted to remain in the Medicare program, he said, it would have to accept "mass regression in the number and quality of services offered the sick and injured."

Valley Baptist is a vital medical facility. It is the primary source of neurosurgery, coronary care, cobalt treatment and radioisotope laboratory services for the more than 400,000 inhabitants of the three-county area it serves, as well as for many of the half-million Mexican citizens who live near the Texas border. The nearest comparable medical center is in Houston, more than 300 miles away. "Ironically, these services are among the things Medicare doesn't pay for," Morrison complains. "Along with emergency, obstetrical and pediatric services, the specialties are loss-producing. Our only practical means of maintaining these facilities financially is to include small amounts in the charges to all our patients. Part of the capital that enables us to add such services and to expand our capacity is obtained this way.

"If Medicare doesn't pay its share of these charges," he explained, "our alternatives are to add their share to the bills of our private-pay patients, or absorb the losses, or abandon our programs of progress, or withdraw from Medicare.

"Neither we nor our private-pay patients can afford to assume these additional costs. Ours is not what is commonly described as an affluent community. Our population consists largely of migrant agricultural workers and senior citizen retirees. Area unemployment averages about 8–10 percent and seasonally rises as high as 20 percent. These are the people on whose shoulders Medicare is placing a burden it should carry itself."

Medicare administrators refuse to pay for that portion of a patient's charge that is used to support hospital facilities that were not used by the covered patient. Hospital administrators argue that charges must frequently include a small portion of the cost for maintaining vital hospital facilities that are not used by all patients, because cost of those services would be prohibitive if costs were not spread out. The simple fact, say the hospital spokesmen, is that *all* patients must help pay for the services, or the hospital will have to cease providing them.

"The necessity for manning O.B.—and other services—around the clock is well established," says H.E. "Sandy" Hamilton, director of New Orleans' famed Ochsner Foundation Hospital. "Apparently not so well established is the actual magnitude of the expense this entails. In order to have one person available for duty 24 hours per day, 7 days a week, you have to hire 4.5 persons—and you have to pay them whether or not there are babies for them to deliver.

Obviously, they can't be used elsewhere when they are not actually delivering babies. If they were, they would not be available during that time to O.B.

" 'Charges related to costs' has a nice sensible sound, and, employed in the proper context, it is sensible. But if each pair of parents had to pay the actual cost of their baby's birth . . . the cost of obstetrics would be prohibitive; yet by charging only a small amount to all patients for its maintenance, this essential—but often idle—service has a relatively reasonable price."

Hamilton also complains that Medicare's refusal to pay the costs of replacing obsolete equipment endangers the level of hospital technology. "In this respect," he said, "America is following in England's footsteps. Like England's program, Medicare pays only for costs of operation. Medical equipment in use in English hospitals is astonishingly obsolete and, of course, the hospitals themselves have been unable to expand—have, in fact, fallen into a state of stagnation and decay. If all my patients were under Medicare, ten years from now Ochsner would be exactly the same as it is today —same size, same capacity, same level of technology, same state of the art."

The Social Security Administration answers that the Medicare program offers liberal depreciation allowances, but hospital administrators maintain that the write-offs merely allow them to maintain the status quo but provide no new funds for expansion and modernization. Wilbur Cohen, former Secretary of Health, Education and Welfare, urged that the problem be met by extending Federal controls to require hospitals to invest depreciation allowances, but investment at available rates would fall far short of providing the necessary funds for updating hospital equipment. There are currently available modern replacements for almost every piece of hospital medical equipment—replacements that are far more effective and often perform functions not previously available with the older units. As a result, the costs are higher.

Hamilton pointed out, for example, that in 1959 Ochsner Hospital was able to buy hospital beds for approximately $150 each. The replacement cost had risen to $500 ten years later. Harry Knickerbocker calculated that to accumulate the $500 for the new bed by investing the depreciation allowances—$15 per year for 10 years —"would require an earning rate in excess of 20 percent compounded annually."

"At this level," he said, "earnings rates entail a much higher risk than most hospitals likely would be willing to accept."

As hospitals continue to lose money by handling Medicare cases, the likelihood increases that more and more will follow the example of Valley Baptist and ask the Social Security Administration to remove them from the list of hospitals available to the aged who rely on Medicare for their medical services.

The effects of Medicare have been felt in other ways as well.

In 1961, the small community of Gardner, Kansas, built a new hospital and converted the previous structure into an extended care facility for long-term custodial patients—usually the helpless aged, most of whom needed minor but frequent attention. Gardner put its all into fixing up the "new" facility. Oxygen therapy was available; laboratory facilities were available; emergency drugs and prescription drugs were available; a registered nurse was on duty eight hours a day, supervising a staff of nurses' aides; a doctor made rounds daily. Instead of providing merely another nursing home, Gardner had provided an extended care *hospital*.

Rates were fixed to cover costs, and physician services were provided free. In fact, wrote Dr. A.S. Reece, a Gardner physician, "the only people who made money on this project were the employees serving the patient, [and] the grocer, the milkman and the laundry. Since the drug store was part of the Gardner Community Medical Center that maintained this ECF, its profits were used to help maintain the facility. Routine lab work for diabetics and anemic cases was done without extra charge."

For a rural community in a predominantly rural state, Gardner was doing a good job of meeting its medical problems. The community had a hospital, an extended care facility, a pharmacy, physicians and dentists, nearly all under a single roof. Gardner even had a top-notch ambulance service. "Then," said Dr. Reece, "Medicare came along and this community that was providing high quality, equal service to all its patients, suddenly had expensive, chaotic, controversial, lower quality medicine."

This is what happened to the extended care facility of which the citizens of Gardner, Kansas, had been so proud:

—Funeral home directors, who had been providing the community's ambulance service, found themselves faced with a brace of Medicare requirements. Compliance would have forced the ambulance operators to charge approximately $60 a trip, even if only around a city block. So the ambulance service was discontinued. "Since then," writes Dr. Reece, "our ambulance service has been haphazard and inefficient. Our ambulances are now handled by willing but untrained volunteers. Recently an ambulance was so long getting to a patient that neighbors brought the patient to the hospital in the back end of a pick-up truck. He was dead on arrival."

—Medicare ruled that separate managements would have to be set up for the ECF and the community hospital.

—Another rule required that RNs be on duty in the building 24 hours a day, seven days a week.

—Building codes were changed.

"Even though we had kept up with the building code in regard to old buildings—sprinkler system, emergency water hoses, fire extinguishers—none of this applied to *hospitals* under the new codes," Dr. Reece complained. "The Board of Health tried to figure some way our institution could be classified as a nursing home. But it would have to be classified as a *new* nursing home and, therefore, we would have to have a *new* building."

Managers of the facility decided not to join Medicare. To follow the system's bureaucratic regulations "would have put us in the same position as the ambulance service. The cost would be so great that the patient would be worse off financially, for Medicare would only pay for 100 days; most of these patients were hospitalized for one to 10 years."

But it is frequently not easy to remain out of the Medicare program. Patients and their relatives began to ask why they could not receive Medicare benefits; they were paying the dues for Part "B" (supplementary benefits) and not getting any service in return. The community's doctors worked out a unique plan to help their patients qualify for Medicare benefits: A doctor was calling each day on the patients in the extended care facility. The visit was free, but if the doctor charged, Medicare would pay the fee. So the ECF double-room charge was reduced from $300 a month to $250 a month, and the remaining $50 was rebilled as a physician fee (10 calls a month at $5 each). Thus the patients were able to receive some of the Medicare benefits they were paying for in the form of the lower room charge.

"Since the whole Medical center was subsidized by the physicians," Dr. Reece wrote, "any losses sustained were made up in rental charges to the physicians. The loss sustained in operating the ECF was considerably more than the $50 a month charged for physician services and the doctors paid back these fees, and more too, in the form of rent. Instead of getting rich, our doctors were suffering a *loss*."

But the solution was only temporary. The Kansas State Board of Health, basing its regulations on Medicare standards, refused to re-license the facility unless registered nurses were provided in the building 24 hours a day, every day. "Even if we could have found the RNs," Dr. Reece complains, "this rule would have cost each patient at least $100 a month more, and would not have improved our care or services one bit." The facility's one RN was in the building eight hours a day and at her home, a block away, most of the time she was not at work. In addition, nurses' aides were on duty at all hours.

Meanwhile, Medicare ruled that the patients did not need ten physician visits a month (less than three a week) and allowed payment for only three visits a month—compared with one call every day before Medicare. "Note the inconsistency of these two branches of government," says Dr. Reece, "one insisting that RNs be on duty 24 hours a day, the other claiming that a physician's services were not necessary but three times a month."

Gardner was forced to close the extended care facility of which it had been so proud. Ironically, a majority of the patients went to a brand-new Medicare-approved nursing home that, in keeping with Medicare's *nursing home* regulations, had *no* RNs at all. And, writes Dr. Reece, "it was 14 miles from any MD."

The losers, as always, were the patients.

"We in the Gardner community tried to give . . . the best economical care we could," Dr. Reece said. "Government did not add a thing to medical care in Gardner—it served only to take away the care our patients were already getting."

Medicare has been more than a failure; it has been a *costly* failure. Medicare's financial experience has been one of constant actuarial error. According to Robert J. Myers, for 23 years the chief actuary of the Social Security Administration and now a Professor of Actuarial Science at Temple University, disbursements for hospital insurance benefit payments and administrative expenses for the first three years of the program were $11.2 billion higher than the original estimates—an overrun of more than 41 percent.

When the Medicare program began in July, 1966, government actuaries estimated the 1970 cost of the hospital insurance portion (Part A) at $3.1 billion. When 1970 actually arrived, the costs were nearly double what had been predicted. The cost of the supplementary plan, for payment of doctors' bills, had risen from $623 million a year in fiscal 1967 to an estimated $1.2 billion in fiscal 1971.

Part B premiums and the deductible provision of Part A have shown a corresponding increase. The deductible, which began at $40 in 1966, with a planned gradual escalation, had actually increased a full 50 percent to $60 by 1971. Monthly premiums paid by the aged for supplementary Medicare benefits (primarily professional service fees) rose from $3 a month in 1966 to $4 in 1968 and to $5.60 in 1971. The latest (1970–71) increase, which will cost 19.5 million Medicare subscribers six percent more per month, will cost the nation's general revenues—meaning the nation's taxpayers—an additional $70 million a year in matching funds.

Government medicine has been tried in America—in the VA and county government hospitals, in the Medicaid and Medicare programs. It has compiled a record of consistent failure—a record so clear that one can only conclude that the fault lies in the nature of government health programs themselves. Medicare is, in effect, a trial run for national health insurance. It *is* national health insurance for 10 percent of the nation's population. Those who advocate extending the program to all Americans should heed carefully the lessons of the Medicare experience.

PART FOUR

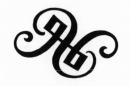

THE CHOICES

15. Problem Solving

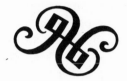

While it is the premise of this book that the presence of a medical or health care "crisis" in the United States is a politically perpetuated myth, there is no denying that those who provide medical care to the American people have problems to solve.

While it is the thesis of this book that national health insurance does not offer viable solutions to those problems, and would likely create extensive new problems in terms of both care and cost, it is nonetheless true that there *is* a need to find solutions.

The solutions, however, lie in the direction of freedom, not compulsion; individual initiative, not governmental regulation; private practice, not government medicine. To the credit of the free market system and the physicians who serve in it, private practitioners themselves have begun to open the doors to major improvements in health care.

The problems, of course, are obvious—particularly to the physician who must live and work with them. While politicians often seek simplistic, politically attractive "answers" (for example, "free" medical care), the doctor must find solutions that will work; he must find them because the welfare of his patients and the quality of his practice depends on the answers he finds. For example, while the average physician bristles under the politically motivated charges of legislators who would attempt to saddle him with the blame for rising health care costs (which are more truthfully attributable to inflationary government policies, union-and-government-forced wage increases, technological advances, and overutilization resulting from Federal and state health programs), he accepts the task of *reducing* care costs because he recognizes that (a) he is better qualified than the average politician or bureaucrat to devise lower-cost care methods, and (b) the welfare of his patients may often depend on the financial feasibility of his proposed treatment.

By the same token, while physician-to-population ratios and the rapid increase in numbers of health care personnel belie the assertions that the nation faces a medical manpower "crisis," the physician, even more than the politician, recognizes the desirability—and sometimes the need—to have more doctors in patient-oriented practices, particularly in rural areas and the core areas of major cities. Again, the doctor assumes the responsibility for producing more doctors because (a) he is better qualified to recognize the true need and the best means of filling the gaps, and (b) excessive demands on his time lessen the time he can give each patient and severely curtail the amount of free time available to him for study, relaxation and family life.

It is obviously impossible to document all of the economies and new programs devised by 300,000-plus physicians to improve the quality of patient care and reduce its cost. A few examples, however, will serve to illustrate the vigor with which the private physician has moved to meet the challenges posed by financial inflation and a growing population.

—Two private practitioners in Phoenix, anesthesiologists John Ford and Wallace Reed, shared a mutual concern: patients who needed only minor surgery, followed by relatively short recuperative periods, were unnecessarily forced to pay for expensive overnight hospitalization and were, at the same time, using hospital beds that might otherwise be available for more seriously ill patients. Ford and Reed decided to do something about it. Investing approximately $400,000 of private capital, they introduced a new concept in surgical treatment—the Surgicenter, an independent, short-stay surgery hospital.

The Surgicenter was opened in 1970, in a gleaming one-story modern building, sandwiched between a church and neighborhood shops. The center contains four operating rooms, a 12-bed recovery room, and ancillary facilities including emergency resuscitation equipment. In addition, Ford and Reed maintain transfer agreements with two hospitals, in case of emergencies that cannot be handled at the Surgicenter. One major hospital, Good Samaritan, is located across the street.

Ambulatory surgical patients who use the center do not have to pay for hospital overhead or share in the costs of 24-hour service that are normally added to a hospital's bill. By the beginning of 1971, 135 Phoenix surgeons had performed operations in the new center. The Surgicenter had already saved patients $180,000, primarily through money saved on hospital-room charges and operating-room fees.

—A similar problem had confronted doctors in Long Beach, California, the year before: short-term patients, who had to be hospitalized to meet insurance reimbursement requirements, were forced to pay hospitalization costs for their recuperation and, in addition, were using bed space that doctors wanted to have available for patients with more serious conditions.

Although regional differences tend to be minimized in professional groups, in which members share common concerns wherever they live, citizens in the Western states seem more willing to look to themselves for answers to their problems, rather than entrusting governments to relieve them of that burden. This is a habit that is probably due at least as much to a distrust of government's abilities as to a tradition of individual self-sufficiency. Thus, rather than crying for Federal funds for their patients, or for Federal aid to their hospitals, the doctors began to search for the answers themselves. The result was a unique day-care facility for short-term recuperative patients. Patients who require only minimal hospitalization, usually to recuperate briefly after diagnostic and therapeutic procedures, are now placed in the day-care unit at Long Beach Memorial Hospital, released the same evening, and billed only $18 for use of the facilities.

What is more, the 12 beds currently in the unit are all in private rooms, each with wall-to-wall carpeting, colorful wall coverings, hot and cold running water, television, wood appointments, a window with an attractive view, electrically operated bed, electronic intercom connection with a central nursing station, high quality food, and care by a registered nurse and a licensed vocational nurse.

In case of an emergency, the patient is just down the corridor from the hospital's surgery, pathology and radiology departments, around the corner from an emergency room, and about a minute away from intensive- or acute-care facilities. In other words, the patient enjoys all of the conveniences of regular hospitalization, but at a savings of from $30 to $50 for the day.

The solution was fairly simple:

(a) Rooms in the new unit are smaller, because there is no need to wheel in gurneys and equipment; thus the hospital saves on both construction and upkeep.

(b) There is no need for the large (and expensive) staff of nurses and paramedical personnel that is required to man adequately other parts of the hospital.

Patients who require 11 hours or less of hospitalization thus benefit financially, while patients who require hospitalization for elective surgery often find the normal wait of a few weeks reduced only to days, because short-term patients are no longer occupying the beds they need.

"The whole project is a splendid example of private practice being able to solve the problems at less cost and with better quality than government could," boasts Dr. Philip Voigt, who was chairman of the hospital medical staff's emergency room committee when it laid the groundwork for the day-care unit in 1969.

"We doctors who are in private practice and who deal with the problems on a day-to-day basis are concerned with financial problems as well as medical care," he said.

"Without the private practice relationship between doctor and patient, this type of unit might not have been developed in our community. A private physician gets much closer to his patients than a government physician. Patients tell us about the burden of their expenses but a government doctor with a county patient may not care about how the bills are paid."

Dr. Padraig Carney, deputy chief of the hospital staff, claims the low cost of the day-care unit also makes it possible for doctors—who would otherwise perform minor procedures in their offices to save patients money—to perform those procedures in the hospital, where staff and equipment make it "easier and safer to treat and observe patients."

When the hospital opened the day-care unit in July, 1970, it was available to patients on a tentative five-day-a-week basis. By that fall, the facility was being used from 7 AM to 6 PM, six days a week. Among the procedures for which patients may recuperate in the day-care unit—for $18—are spinal puncture, sternal puncture, paracentesis/thoracentesis, laryngoscopy/bronchoscopy, anoscopy/sigmoidoscopy, radiological procedures, I.V. cholangiography, IVP, angiography, pneumoencephalography radiation therapy, phlebotomy, blood transfusions, post-recovery phase following closed reduction or open reduction treatment of fractures, and the post-recovery phase of minor surgeries such as D&C.

—Four years earlier, doctors opened an 86-bed advanced-care unit at the Long Beach Medical Center. The special facility provides recuperative beds for patients who have passed through the acute phase in their recovery from heart attacks, strokes, serious fractures, and other injuries or illness that require them to remain hospitalized or to receive rehabilitation, but who no longer need as much nursing care and paramedical support service as that provided in typical hospital facilities. Like the day-care center, the advanced-care facility includes a large number of luxuries, including ice-water taps and coffee in each room; a color television lounge; and a landscaped courtyard with benches, a waterfall and radiant heating under walkways.

The advanced-care facility has been cited by the Kellogg Foundation for saving a quarter of a million dollars a year. Patients in the unit pay one-fourth less than they would if they remained in typical hospital surroundings.

—Unlike government health service physicians, and physicians in large pre-payment practices, who frequently serve their patients on a 9-to5 basis, five private practitioners in Tell City, Indiana, near the Kentucky and Ohio borders, decided on their own to extend service to their townspeople by building a new clinic and working out schedules to keep the clinic open, with at least one of the five on duty, 24 hours a day, seven days a week.

—In an attempt to increase the number of doctors available to see patients, physicians dig deeply into their own pockets. In mid-1971, the American Medical Association announced that in the previous nine years the AMA had guaranteed $48 million in loans to medical students, and had given another $50 million to the nation's medical schools. At the time of the report, there were more

than 7,500 students either in medical school or serving in internship or residency programs with the help of loans guaranteed by the
AMA.

—At the same time, largely through the impetus of private physicians, a number of the nation's leading medical schools have turned
actively to a new emphasis on motivating students to serve in patient-oriented care.

Dr. Walter C. Bornemeier, president of the AMA from mid-
1970 until mid-1971, has pointed out that much of the reason for
the shortage of practicing doctors in some areas is attributable to
the government itself, a conclusion shared by Washington columnist Allan C. Brownfeld. "Government, rather than assisting in
eliminating the doctor shortage, has been one of the major con-
tributors to it," Brownfeld wrote in the December 26, 1970, issue
of *Human Events.*

The problem began in the late 1950s when Congress, under the
prodding of the influential Mary Lasker and research-minded Senator Lister Hill, began to appropriate far more for medical research
than the medical profession could then accommodate. As a result,
it became necessary to train new researchers, and young doctors
were persuaded to extend their training into this area rather than
enter patient-oriented practice. As the trend mounted, medical
schools, seeking ways to accommodate the sudden influx of Federal
money, began to set aside large areas for research laboratories,
making less space available for the teaching of students.

In addition, recent trends toward specialization have removed
many thousands of doctors from patient care for an additional two
to five years, and have resulted in fewer doctors—when they reach
practice—being available for the general-practice responsibilities at
the entry point into the medical system. At the beginning of 1971,
there were approximately 35,000 doctors in specialty training, plus
5,000 who had quit practice to teach in hospitals, and another
10–12,000 working as full-time medical school instructors. These
three sources alone, exclusive of the doctors who had gone into
research, accounted for more than 50,000 doctors removed from
the actual care of patients.

Obviously the problem begins in the medical schools. And it is
there that the profession is moving to halt the problem. While the
government has often served only to compound the drift away from

practice, doctors themselves are moving now to straighten things out.

—What may be the prime example predates the problem by a number of years. Since 1931, private practitioners in Durham, North Carolina, have been contributing a good part of the fee income they receive for in-hospital service to the development of the Duke University Medical Center and to the teaching of private medical practice in the University's hospital.

The Duke Medical Center includes a private-practice clinic (known as the Private Diagnostic Clinic) that provides support personnel—including receptionists, nurses, business staff, messengers and laboratory technicians—for a number of private doctors who treat their ambulatory patients in the clinic. These doctors admit their patients who need hospitalization to the University Hospital, in which they, as senior staff members, teach the private practice of medicine, including specialties in surgery, medicine, obstetrics and gynecology, ophthalmology, pediatrics and psychiatry.

Patients are charged a professional fee, commensurate with standard fees in the area, but the money received is shared with the university, with the university getting the lion's share. Although the distribution pattern varies, Dr. Morton D. Bogdonoff, writing in a 1969 issue of *Archives of Internal Medicine*, reported that at that time doctors were keeping 47 percent or less of the fees collected in the Department of Medicine. Of the remainder, approximately 25 percent was used to cover the overhead costs of the clinic and office operation, 15 to 20 percent was allocated for development of the department, and eight percent was placed in a general building fund.

The Duke Medical Center, like most others, has accepted Federal funds for expansion, and through that means has added basic science facilities, clinical research areas, public ambulatory clinics, laboratories, and radiologic study areas, and has renovated hospital wards. All of the matching money—the funds that had to be put up by local sources to match the Federal grants—came from the general building fund developed through the fee contributions of the private doctors.

—"The patient does not wish to be treated as a statistic from a group approach, but as an individual—a person . . . The emphasis in the educational program should be on the individual—whether he be student, patient, or physician-teacher."

The speaker was Dr. George T. Harrell, who was being interviewed by reporter William Ecenbarger for *Private Practice*. Dr. Harrell had recently become Dean of Pennsylvania State University's new College of Medicine in the small town of Hershey.

Even among members of the medical profession, Hershey was better known in 1969 for the chocolate bars manufactured there than for the medical school that had moved to town. Today that has changed. The Hershey Medical School, as it has come to be known, has caught the profession's attention with its attempts to turn out *practicing* doctors. To carry out Dr. Harrell's philosophy, each student is assigned to a local family that is under the care of one of the five family physicians in the school's Department of Family and Community Medicine, itself a fairly new teaching concept. "For his entire four years of medical education," reports Ecenbarger, "the student will be on hand for every office visit, house call or hospital admission involving any member of the assigned family."

The purpose is to teach students to care for the daily, routine illnesses that make up the bulk of a practitioner's work, rather than placing overemphasis on the more serious, but less frequent, cases that take up a specialist's time and frequently result in a patient being admitted to a hospital. In addition to helping increase the supply of doctors in actual practice, Harrell hopes to inculcate the habit of treating patients while they are ambulatory, thus greatly reducing health care costs. "We want to head off illness before it results in a trip to the hospital, where the real costs of medicine are incurred today," he says.

—The developments at Hershey are part of a continuing trend toward a re-establishment of medical schools as centers for the teaching of practice-oriented doctors. Departments of Family Practice are beginning to spring up, from the Medical College of South Carolina, in Charleston, to the University of California's medical school campus in Loma Linda. The American Medical Association has advanced general practice, with a few modifications, to a new specialty known as family practice, and residents in that field are now in some of the nation's hospitals.

In short, while the Federal Government has contributed largely to the drawing of medical students *from* patient care, the medical profession has been trying to draw more and more young people into medical schools and then into patient care.

Ironically, in an age of extensive "social awareness," doctors are forced to fight another major rival for the attention of the young physicians they have educated to care for the sick. That rival is the so-called social awareness, itself. An Associated Press survey in 1970 revealed that none of the 42 interns and residents at one Boston hospital planned to enter private practice. A survey of graduating seniors at three Boston medical schools failed to turn up a single student who intended to enter private practice. The reason is distressingly simple: liberal academicians and politicians are calling on medical students to "become involved" in the larger world about them. Such influences have so infused today's medical students (and other students as well) with a crusading zeal to help The People, that they have no time to spare for the individual people who need their help.

"I would like to solve social problems myself," Dr. Michael Halberstam, a Washington, D.C., internist, wrote in the *New York Times Magazine*; "but while I did, who'd be minding the store? If physicians are to be trained to 'alter and alleviate' social conditions, why did I bother to study anatomy, which really was sort of a drag? . . .

"I would guess that my black patients care less about my social and political feelings than my ability to diagnose chest pain and my availability on a Sunday afternoon . . .

"Each doctor testifying before Congress, writing articles, lobbying for gun control, marching for peace in Vietnam, or distributing petitions to abolish the Supreme Court," he said, "is a doctor away from his patients or his research."

The call for doctor "involvement" often comes from the same activists who denounce the medical profession for a doctor shortage and insist on new Federal health programs to revamp the medical care system. For example, Dr. Richard Kunnes, who led the disruptive march on the American Medical Association's 1969 convention, has admitted that he does not intend to enter practice. Yet the profession continues to increase the number of doctors available to care for the sick—an increase of 28 percent in 11 years, while the nation's population was growing only 12 percent.

—Doctors themselves have been instrumental in a move to use

returning military corpsmen to ease their patient loads. Although many doctors are reluctant to hire the corpsmen, realizing the danger of legal liability if a non-physician employee makes an error that results in harm to a patient, many others are experimenting with the idea. For example, the Washington State Medical Society has cooperated in the enrollment of former corpsmen in a three-month training program, and the state's rural doctors have taken the corpsmen under their wings for year-long apprenticeships, after which it is planned that the doctors will hire the corpsmen to assist in treating infections, lacerations, moderate traumas, and other illnesses or injuries, and, at times, to serve as surgical assistants—all to free the doctor for more patient care.

Dr. Richard Bunch, a general practitioner in Othello, Washington, has estimated that use of the corpsmen will permit doctors such as himself to see up to 20 additional patients a day.

—Although pre-payment group practices have many drawbacks, particularly in loss of the personal relationship between doctor and patient, and overdemand for care, causing insufficient time for treatment of those who actually need care the most (see Chapter 7), they have some advantages as well.

The Kaiser Foundation Health Plan, a pre-payment program established purely as a private enterprise venture, has some two million subscribers after 26 years, and in some cases provides care for less than private care on a fee-for-service basis. As an example, at the end of 1970, a family of three or more, enrolled under a typical Kaiser plan, paid a fee of $35.40 a month for hospitalization up to 111 days a year, office treatment (which cost $1 a visit, in addition to the pre-payment) house calls (an additional $5), and all surgery, X-rays, laboratory tests, and maternity care (which might range in cost from nothing to $100, depending on the plan).

For many Americans the total cost of approximately $425 a year (assuming no maternity care) is considerably more than they would ordinarily pay through the fee-for-service system. But for a family that encounters a great deal of sickness in a year, the program could be financially beneficial.

The Kaiser plan is operated totally within the context of the private enterprise system, and without government involvement. Similar programs have been undertaken by private companies in other parts of the country. From the Surgicenter in Phoenix to the

24-hour-a-day, everyday, clinic in Tell City, Indiana; from the Kaiser pre-payment plan in five states to the day-care unit in Long Beach and the medical corpsmen in Washington State, private doctors and private enterprise are developing programs to attempt to provide better care at lower cost.

Governments have failed miserably in their efforts to provide good health care in this country and throughout Europe. It is becoming increasingly clear that the road to a constantly improving medical system lies through a *removal* of the fetters of bureaucracy, and increased reliance on the industry and initiative of private industry and the medical profession itself.

16. The Right to Health Care

Throughout most of this book we have been discussing the *practical* effects of national health programs: what such programs would cost and how they would affect the quality of medical care available to you and your family; we have been discussing whether such a program would work (that is, whether it would accomplish the goals its sponsors envision) and whether what we received would be worth the price we would have to pay for it.

But national health insurance is more than a pragmatic political issue; the debate over government-funded medical care encompasses basic philosophies of government and the proper role of government in a free society. The debate may ultimately be resolved—politically—on pragmatic grounds alone, but the society must some day confront the more basic issues—such issues as:

(a) When may government properly take the property of its citizens for the use of society or other citizens?

(b) When may government properly deprive a citizen of the right to bargain for an acceptable compensation for his services?

(c) When may a nation's government properly regulate the activities of that nation's citizens?

Each of these issues is vital to the consideration of any program of national health insurance, for if government, to support such a program, improperly seizes the property of its citizens (through taxation), or unjustly deprives a citizen of the right to sell his services at an agreed-upon price, then the issue properly becomes one not merely of workability but of right and wrong.

The basic premise underlying the argument for "free" medicine may be simply stated: each citizen, the health planner will say, has a "right" to good health. It thus follows, according to the planners' equation, that because sickness or injury deprive a citizen of his right to be healthy, he has a presumptive right to be made well. From that presumption it follows that if one has a right to be healthy, and a further right to be restored to health if that health is impaired by injury or illness, he should not be denied complete and ready access to that care due to his inability to pay its provider, or due to failures of the system to make such care easily available.

On its face, both the premise and the conclusions sound reasonable enough. After all, is it not desirable that each citizen should have both good health and adequate care to maintain that health? The answer, of course, is "yes." And because the answer is "yes," there too seldom is argument with the thesis that follows—the thesis that each citizen shall, as a matter of right, be *provided* that health care by the society, through its government. We have, after all, agreed that the availability of universal health care is a desirable goal. This, however, evades two necessary questions: (1) does national health insurance, or government-funded health care, offer the best means of attaining that goal?, and (2) does the "desirability" of such an end make proper the means by which it is sought?

The first question is answered in the preceding 15 chapters; the evidence seems clearly to indicate that government health care programs are insufficient to achieve the goals of providing either universal care or reasonably adequate care.

The second question is the subject of this chapter. My answer to it is: "No; the fact that an end is desirable does not justify the use of ethically improper means to attain that end." That being the case, it becomes necessary to determine whether or not the means by which the planners would provide health care to each citizen (national health insurance) is a proper and ethical function of government. I submit that it is not.

Good health is a right, but in one sense only: as one may not, without legal authority, take the life of another, neither may one harm the health of another. There is ample legal precedent to affirm this right of each citizen to be held safe against intentional or careless harm to either his physical or mental health. But it is important to delineate the boundaries of that right. If one citizen (John Doe) harms another citizen (Richard Roe), then the injured party (Roe) has a right to seek redress against the man who injured him. That, however, is as far as Roe's rights go (except, in a purely legal sense, in cases of vicarious liability). Rights are essentially negative in character: they are guarantors against an action by another. The right to live, for example, is the right not to be deprived of life by another, and its corollary, the right to pursue those actions that sustain life, is actually the right not to be harmed or interfered with in that pursuit.

When the promoters of government health programs argue that health *care* is a right, they seek to go one step further—to enforce that "right" against innocent parties (in the case of national health insurance, against the physician and the society, as I shall show). These "rights" would not merely guarantee Roe that he would not be harmed, they would confer on him the "right" to force Doe to take positive action to benefit Roe. Under such a program, if Roe were to fall ill from no discoverable human cause—that is, if he were to contract a case of measles, suffer a heart attack, fall asleep at the wheel of his automobile, or develop a cancer—his "right" to health would be presumed to be violated. He would be presumed to have a proper "claim" against society for the restoration of his health. Since society is not an entity in itself, but only a conglomerate of separate, individual, entities (its citizens), the claim against society would necessarily be made against the only persons in that society who would be capable of "paying" it—(a) a doctor, or an entire staff of medical personnel, and (b) each individual taxpayer, who would be called upon to pay the bills incurred in restoring, or trying to restore, Roe's health.

In other words, Roe's presumed "right" to health care would give him the power to force another person to confer benefits on him (that is, it would give the government power to exert such force, in Roe's name). For example, a doctor would be required, under national health insurance, to devote his time and effort, and the knowledge acquired through strenuous activity and personal sacrifice, to care for Roe whether he chose to do so or not (under those systems in which physicians are assigned responsibility for patients in a designated area or facility). Or he would be required to use that time, effort and knowledge in Roe's behalf for whatever compensation the government saw fit to bestow (under *any* system of national health insurance, with its ultimate control of fees).

Does the "desirability" of Roe's good health properly give him the right to maintain that health by forcing others to do his bidding? I maintain that it does not. Such a concept would have no logical end (although limits would be arbitrarily set, and continually revised). For example, it is also clearly desirable that each person have food, clothing and shelter. If desirability were the applicable criterion, it would be ethically proper for government to force each working citizen (through taxation) to provide food, clothing and shelter for those persons who lack them. It is clearly desirable, in an age of sprawling urban communities, that each citizen have an automobile with which to carry groceries from the market, or with which he or she can reach a doctor or hospital in time of need. Using the desirability of mobility as justification, therefore, one can make a case for the use of government force to seize John Doe's income (through taxation) to purchase "free" automobiles for each citizen.

In the above example, the taxpaying citizen has had the rewards for his labor seized to provide an ever-increasing supply of "desirable" or "needed" goods or services. But the "desirability" of a product or service, or the "need" for it, does not provide ethical justification for government provision. To provide the "desirable" or "needed" service or goods to Citizen A, the government has forcibly taken the income of Citizen B and redistributed it. Citizen B is thus an economic slave: that is, although he is not forced by government to work, he must do so to support himself, and is forced by government to surrender a considerable portion of his reward for that work for the use of other citizens. His is not slavery to a single master; he is a slave, economically, to a whole society of slaveholders.

Such a system is a base distortion of the concept of "rights," whether natural or civil. A "right" is defensible at law against willful (and sometimes against accidental) violation. But the defense of that right does not impinge upon the rights of innocent third parties except in prohibiting their violation of another person's rights. For example, citizen A, as a corollary of his birthright to life, has the right to enjoy the fruits of his labors (the means by which he sustains life); thus, he can own property. Citizen B, as a corollary of his birthright of liberty, has the right to move about in freedom—except that he must stop short of trespassing on A's land or stealing A's personal property.

Those who advocate national health insurance (that is, those who advocate governmental regulation of a physician's fees, and distribution and control of his services), seek to justify their action on the basis of "need" for the doctor's services. But the government has no more right to "distribute" a physician's work, or to control his payment for it, than it would have the right to control the labor of a plumber or electrician, both of whom, as free men, sell their services to customers of their own choosing, and work only for those willing to pay an agreed-upon price for the service. Because a physician's labor often involves the preservation of life, the similarity between the doctor and the plumber is often overlooked. The planners contend that the doctor is morally obligated to provide his service because it is more important than the service of a plumber, electrician, or carpenter. In effect, the physician is thus being punished for having chosen to endure the rigorous (and expensive) training required to master his profession. Had he chosen to pursue a less demanding calling—a calling that would have provided fewer benefits to his fellow man—his fellows would not now be demanding the right to control his labor and his income.

Those who rush to preserve the citizen's "right" to health care overlook the legitimate rights of those who must provide that care. It is true that a doctor will often feel an obligation to use his knowledge to help persons regardless of their ability to pay him for his service—but that is a *voluntary* act of charity. He cannot, morally, be *forced* to provide his labor for reduced reward any more than he can be morally forced to surrender his personal property to another, for his knowledge and his skill *are* his personal property —as much so as his home and its furnishings.

To claim that medical *care* is a right—that a man has a right to be cared for—is to presuppose that he is to be taken care of *by somebody.* And the question then becomes: What of that other some-body's rights? That is the flaw in the concept that the citizen has a right to health care; if he is to be cared for by a physician, then what of that physician's rights? As a citizen, the physician, too, must be able to lay claim to protection of his right to his own time and his own labor. Even though many physicians will willingly serve their fellow men at personal sacrifice, it is immoral to assume that they can be *made* to serve, by order of society. Such an order would make slaves of physicians, slaveholders of patients, and slavemasters of the citizenry.

If a doctor is *forced* to practice under a system of national health insurance, he is a slave to his fellow citizens.

If he is given the option of practicing under the system or not practicing at all, he is not a slave, but is being effectively deprived of his right to pursue his profession and sell his services *unless* he accepts slavery.

If he is given the option of practicing under a national health system or remaining in private practice, he is the victim of govern-ment-sponsored unfair competition, for many of his prospective patients, having already paid for medical care through taxation, will choose not to pay again for private care.

But the argument that each citizen has a "right" to health care envisions more than the forced attention—or voluntary attention at forcibly reduced payment—of the medical professional. Each tax-paying citizen will be forced to surrender part of his income to support the system.

If one citizen falls asleep at the wheel of his automobile and finds himself in need of medical care, who will pay for that care? You will.

If another citizen smokes four packages of cigarettes a day, and develops a lung cancer, who will pay for his care? You will.

If a third citizen, financially poor, develops pneumonia and re-quires hospitalization, who will pay for his care? You will.

If a fourth citizen, with a good job and substantial income, is hospitalized for a broken foot, who will pay for his care? You will.

Under the broader programs that have been proposed, you, as a taxpayer, will pay not merely for forced "charity" to the aged or indigent, but for whatever health services are needed or demanded by any citizen, prosperous or poor. And even under the less comprehensive programs, you will provide, through taxation, the general revenue dollars expended to fund the government health systems. You will pay in each of these cases, though you might choose to use the hundreds of dollars the program will cost you for other, personal, needs or desires. You will be providing the "forced labor" to pay for the system, because the wages you earn at your job will be confiscated by the government to pay for the medical care of somebody else. If health care is a right, it must also create a loss of rights.

The provision of government-funded health care is not a proper function of government. Whereas the Constitution grants authority to the national government to promote the *general* welfare, there is no grant of authority by means of which Federal officers may use the funds at their disposal to provide for private benefits to individual citizens.

The story is told that when frontiersman Davy Crockett was a member of the Congress he voted for appropriations to relieve individual distresses, and was promptly upbraided by an irate constituent who praised Crockett for his compassion but challenged the Congressman to find in the Constitution any authority whereby he might spend tax monies taken from other citizens to fulfill his own charitable instincts. Crockett, after studying the Constitution, and being much closer than we are today to the actual events that led to the drafting of that document, concluded that there was indeed no such authority, and resolved thereafter to be charitable only with his own funds or funds he could persuade his colleagues to contribute.

So it is today. While none will deny the desirability of charitable assistance to those who are in need (and, indeed, Americans contribute large amounts each year to help persons less fortunate than themselves), there is no constitutional authorization for the taxing of all citizens—some of whom may be charitably inclined and some of whom may not, or may prefer other charities—to provide government-funded medical services. Nor is there constitutional authority for the Federal Government to tax its citizens for the provision of health care under a theory of service, rather than charity, for the proper services of government are carefully delineated in the Constitution—an instrument designed to preserve individual rights by spelling out limits to the Federal powers.

Dr. Michael P. Hyman, a young Denver physician, summed up the philosophical considerations in an article written while he was editor of the medical-student newsletter at Wayne State University, in Detroit. Although those who claim that health care is a right are undoubtedly men of good will, he wrote, and advocate national health insurance because they believe it is the most direct route toward better health care, "a free society depends on the willingness of men to sometimes forego the most direct route to their goals in exchange for the mutual respect of individual rights which make that free society possible. If man is his brother's keeper, it must be by choice."

The concept of a "right" to free health care—a right to be taken care of—finds much of its support in the more general philosophical attitudes that are prevalent in the society as a whole. As every movement rests on a philosophical base, the movement to create a new state-financed and state-controlled system of medicine rests to a large extent on the philosophical base of existentialism. The dismal philosophies of Dostoevsky, Kafka, Sartre, Camus, Rilke, Heidegger, Jaspers and Kierkegaard have become the basis for the programs that would make physicians employees of the state and guarantee each citizen the right to be cared for at no direct expense to himself. The drive to give free medical care to all is based on the concept that man is a helpless victim of life and must be protected by society. This is also the basic concept of existentialism—a philosophy that views life as hopeless; that views man as alienated, uprooted, helplessly entrapped in circumstance.

This is not a philosophy of the past—it is the basic philosophy of today. One need not read Dostoevsky or Kafka to find it. One need not go back even so far as Camus' *The Stranger*, or Sartre's *The Age of Reason*, both of which were written during the past 30 years. We can find it in today's plays. *Hair* is a good example—Claude, the entrapped and doomed hero, is at one with the entrapped and doomed Meursault in *The Stranger* or the entrapped and doomed Pablo in Sartre's *The Wall*. One can see the same philosophy in today's movies; read it in today's books; hear it in today's music, or in college lectures.

This "modern" philosophy holds that life is a succession of tragedies, or, at best, of meaningless episodes; that the citizen is entrapped in a series of events over which he has no control and which he can only observe from the sidelines—a mere spectator to the determination of his fate. The political extension of this philosophy is based on the conviction that people are victims of circumstance, helpless to prepare for their own well-being; that, therefore, society must protect its citizens against the struggles of life. Not only does existentialism offer a convenient out for wrongs or mistakes ("I couldn't help it"), it also offers a political philosophy: the benevolent government.

Medicine is a natural target for such a political philosophy. In what way are people constantly buffeted by the fates? In matters of health. In what way are people drained of their money? In expenditures to stay well. In what way should government protect its citizens? By demanding that doctors—or other citizens—keep them well. Other solutions—free enterprise medicine, individual apportionment of expenses and savings, private insurance—are not compatible with the current philosophy. Politicians and social planners who start with an existentialist view of life are unable to conceive of man as being capable of meeting life's challenges or providing for his own well-being. Such a thought is not consistent with their basic premises.

There is yet another factor that enters into the willingness of many citizens to appropriate the physician's time and labors for "service" to the community. It is a factor to which the doctor, himself, has contributed.

For years the physician carefully nurtured the image of the old family doctor with sugar pills for the kids and a comforting word for the sick. He was a Rock of Gibraltar and the possessor of enormous supplies of understanding and compassion. He had *help* to offer, not services to sell. If the nineteenth-century doctor conveyed an image, it was that of a devoted humanitarian, a man whose sole *raison d'etre* was to make others well.

Now things have changed. Because science has provided more to work with, today's physician gives injections rather than holding hands; prescribes helpful medicines rather than offering placebos or sitting for long futile hours at a bedside. Yet those same advances that have enabled the physician to do more for his patients have also driven a widening wedge between them. A public that has been conditioned to think of a doctor as a kindly servant, sitting at the bedside, cannot readily adjust to thinking of him as a professional man, scientifically trained, but otherwise much like the man next door: overworked and too busy to give undue compassion to trivial complaints; concerned about paying his own employees and office rent, and providing for his family.

Much of the public—including many persons who normally oppose most forms of government control—is amazingly willing to consider some form of control over the physician. As the doctor once wished, he is thought of as a public servant—one whose sole purpose is to take care of the patient. Obviously, if the patient can find ways to bring this about more "efficiently," or for less personal cost, that's just good business—like buying a more economical automobile. Consequently the patient, in his role as a citizen, finds nothing improper in imposing on the physician controls that he— whether an attorney, plumber, electrician or mechanic—would greatly resist should they be proposed to apply to him.

National health insurance is being offered by politicians and health planners as a means to "systematize" the delivery of health care and provide "free," universally available, care to the American public. Those who oppose national health insurance base their opposition on the question: Will it do what its backers say it will do, and will it do it as cheaply as they say it will? Because this is the sole basis of the debate, those who conclude that a proposed government health plan will *not* fulfill the promises of its sponsors feel no compunction in the offering of alternatives that are distinguished only by detail, and not by concept. The truth is: there is much more than a simple problem of pragmatic politics to be resolved in the formulating of this country's medical-care system. The issue is complex and involves basic philosophical and ethical considerations.

The evidence is clear that national health programs are costly and inefficient, and result in greatly reduced standards of medical care. In short, government medicine does not work. But the question involves far more than that. National health insurance must be rejected not only because it is unworkable, but also because it would, through the imposition of *ersatz* rights, deprive the nation's doctors and its taxpayers of rights that are very real. *Free enterprise* is the moral means of providing health care, because it forces no man to work for any other. It is based, instead, on a basic belief in the ability of most men to regulate their own lives.

17. A Time for Choosing

By the beginning of 1971, a small band of powerful political and labor leaders in this country had begun impatiently to demand a health care revolution. "Today," complained Senator Edward Kennedy, "the United States is the only major industrial nation in the world that does not have a national health service or a program of national health insurance." Ironically, while all this was happening, Britain's Institute of Economic Affairs was releasing a survey which revealed that 70 percent of the British people were unhappy with the medical system that Kennedy and his colleagues seek to emulate.

National health insurance need not come to pass in the United States. Its advocates have proceeded to this point by default, but it is not too late for those who oppose government medical programs to let their views be known. There is ample reason to do so.

The American people do not support national health insurance. Republican Senator Henry Bellmon, whose Oklahoma constituency includes a large number of welfare recipients and whose state is overwhelmingly comprised of Democratic voters, reports that a 1971 survey revealed very little support for national health insurance. About the same time, a survey of its own leadership by the state's Democratic Party, the political base of House Speaker Carl Albert and former Democratic National Chairman Fred Harris, revealed that only about half of the actual party leadership—traditionally more liberal than the average voter—favored such a program. The findings in Oklahoma were borne out by nationwide Harris and Gallup polls, both revealing general public satisfaction with the current medical system.

Politicians who endorse and introduce national health insurance programs hope to use the issue to win the support of the labor voter, inundated with official union propaganda about the alleged "health care crisis" and the need for national health insurance. Even in this fertile field, however, advocates of government health programs are not finding the extensive support they had hoped for: the American Medical Association, on June 1, 1971, reported that a survey by a major national union had revealed some 40 percent of the membership opposed to the Kennedy bill (which had been endorsed by the United Auto Workers and the AFL-CIO). The truth of the matter is, the public simply is not excited about national health insurance. Senator Bellmon has told friends privately that the issue has not generated any significant mail from constituents. Dr. Leona Baumgartner, Executive Director of the Tri-State Regional Medical Program (for Massachusetts, New Hampshire and Rhode Island), and an outspoken critic of private medicine, admitted in a 1969 speech to the American Academy of Pediatrics that "neither the doctor *nor his patient* . . . seem to have any real motivation . . . for changing things . . ." (emphasis added).

The reason, simply, is that there is no need for an expensive and controversial new health care system.

Much of the campaign for national health insurance is conducted through newspaper articles, speeches (with no opportunities for questions afterwards) and interviews by newsmen friendly to the cause. Therefore, there is seldom a challenge to any of the principal assertions of the planners—assertions I have challenged in this book. Statements that American health care is inferior (statements supported only by the demonstrably false use of non-comparable infant mortality figures) are passed on to the public and repeated unquestioningly by speakers at every level; statements that health care costs are out of line with other costs, and that Americans cannot afford to stay well—statements belied both by economic truths and by the general health of the public—are unquestioned.

Occasionally, however, a proponent of national health insurance will participate in a debate, or in a question-and-answer session, with interesting results. Invariably, when allegations about health care are refuted, the argument becomes: "But the *poor* do not have access to this care." Similarly, when allegations that costs have made health care inaccessible are refuted, the argument again becomes: "But the *poor* have no insurance and cannot afford the care."

Advocates of national health insurance, it seems, would force every American into a quasi-socialized medical system—a system that would cost the average worker more than twice what he now pays for all health care, and that would force him into massive health centers, with loss of privacy and a loss of personal relationship with his doctor—to provide a new health program to care for the 11 percent of the under-65 population that is not covered by private health insurance.

This raises two important questions:

First, is national health insurance a viable solution to the problem of providing adequate care for the poor and the aged?

Second, why is national health insurance proposed for all Americans, including those who *do* have access to good medical care at a price they can afford to pay?

To answer the first question, we must first concede that the aged, of course, have more need for medical attention (the poor do also, but largely due to non-medical factors such as malnutrition, poor housing, etc.). Also, by definition, the poor are unable to pay for care that is not donated to them (and, likewise, the elderly are generally less well-off financially than younger persons). Yet there is ample evidence that the private medical system has taken care of these problems in an imperfect but reasonably successful manner: the aged, too, have longer life expectancies at every age than in the past, and the poor (that is, blacks, the only "poor" for whom accurate statistics are available) also have increased life expectancies and reduced mortality rates in infancy and at every age, and at some ages have longer life expectancies than whites. (See Chapter 4 for a more detailed presentation.)

The question then becomes: Can national health insurance do a *better* job? Obviously, the proposition that national health insurance will work is disproved by the assertion of its need.

The Federal Government now spends in excess of $18 billion a year for hospital care, yet we are told that the nation is in the midst of a health care "crisis." Why? For the last six years, the elderly and the poor *have been* enrolled in programs of national health insurance: Medicare for the aged and Medicaid (in addition to state welfare programs) for the indigent. The United States taxpayers have spent billions of dollars in this time to support programs passed specifically for the purpose of making health care accessible to the persons whom advocates of *total* national health insurance now contend are most in need of improved medical care.

If Medicare and Medicaid have worked, there is no need for further government programs to help the aged and the poor. But if they have not worked—as they *obviously* have not—it is clear that government health programs do not work; they merely drain the taxpayers, restrict medical care, and intrude on the privacy of those unfortunate persons who are subject to such a system.

This brings us to the second question: Why is national health insurance proposed for everyone? Why does Senator Kennedy propose a compulsory government program under which the working man with limited income would be taxed to pay for the medical care not only of himself and his neighbors, but also of the J. Paul Gettys, H. L. Hunts, Nelson Rockefellers and Edward Kennedys? Why does President Nixon propose a health program that would require employers to pay most of the health insurance premiums for employees who are, in most cases, making wages that permit them to insure themselves?

The answer has its roots not in medicine but in politics and in social philosophy. It seems apparent that the advocates of national health insurance seek not a medical goal but a philosophical or social goal. Those who urge a medical revolution—who urge us to destroy our free-enterprise medical system and replace it with government health programs—are closing their eyes to the failures of government medicine in this country and elsewhere. Their crusade is based not so much in criticism of the results of free-enterprise medicine as in the philosophical conviction that another form of social system is preferable to free enterprise. They believe it is proper for the state to provide for the individual; they believe it is proper for the state to control, finance and direct the major areas of activity within the nation, whether that activity be public or private.

To test the validity of this assertion, one can consider the identity

of the major promoters of national health insurance programs. With
the exceptions of the American Medical Association and the Nixon
administration, most of the leading advocates of the "medical revolution" are persons who have long favored, and who continue to
advocate, increased Federal participation in *many* sectors. In fact,
the Committee for National Health Insurance—the Reuther Committee—consists primarily of those same persons who have for
years championed increased governmental regulation and direction. (The AMA proposed its own plan because it fears that some
plan might be passed, and wants to have some voice in shaping
whatever law might eventually materialize; some within the Nixon
administration admit candidly that the President has proposed his
own plan because he felt it politically necessary to prevent Democrats from pre-empting what might well be a major issue in the
1972 elections.)

The campaign for national health insurance has not arisen spon-
taneously, in reaction to any so-called "health care crisis"; as I
demonstrate in Appendix I, it is the result of a long and patient
drive. And the planners now see their goal but a short distance
away.

It is not too late to stop them.

There is no medical crisis in the United States, but there may be
one soon. Experience with government health programs in this
country and elsewhere makes it ominously clear that a national
health insurance program may well result in a severe doctor shortage, overcrowding of hospitals and physicians' offices, long waiting
lists for hospital care, inadequate facilities, loss of privacy, Federal
bankruptcy, and, eventually perhaps, discussion in this nation of the
need for mercy killings of the aged to reduce the unbearable costs
of government medicine.

The choice before us is simple. You and I are now covered by
private health plans and we are familiar with them; we know what
they provide and what they cost, and we know the agent who
services them. We know our doctors and most of us have confidence in them. We are reasonably healthy, for the most part, and
save for an occasional serious illness or injury, most of us pay a
relatively small part of our incomes to stay well.

National health insurance will destroy private insurance in the
United States. In return, its advocates promise to solve a fictional

health crisis. But we might well ask: "Can national health insurance even solve the problems that admittedly do exist?" Government has made similar promises in the past: it has promised to solve the problems of agriculture, of housing, of welfare. Instead, government intervention has compounded the problems. Do you and I want to spend from $12 to $80 billion a year to replace private medical care with government medical programs that have failed wherever they have been tried?

Fortunately, politicians react to pressure from the voters. If we do not want to sacrifice private medical care to the ambitious dreams of the planners, we can still do something about it. The planners are few; we, the voters, are many. Our letters, our protests, can prevent the enactment of expensive and disastrous government health schemes. But only if we act soon.

The propagandists for national health insurance have leveled their attacks on your doctor and on his system of private medical care. But if national health insurance is enacted, it will be you, the patient, who will be the victim.

Appendix I.
A History of the Campaign for National Health Insurance

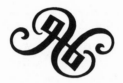

"The idea of national health insurance is an idea whose time has come," Representative Richard Fulton said recently. "The question is what plan? And when can we develop one that works?"

But national health insurance plans are nothing new; they have been proposed, debated, and tried—unsuccessfully—for nearly 300 years. The answer to Fulton's question—when can we develop a plan that works?—has eluded social planners since the sixteenth century, when Queen Elizabeth I proposed a vague "Poor Law" that produced few noticeable results.

Hugh Chamberlain, a member of the British Parliament, was the first politician to decide that national health insurance was "an idea whose time had come"—in 1689, when he proposed a comprehensive government health insurance program (much like today's Kennedy plan) whereby "care might be taken that all sick, as well poor as rich, shall be advised and visited when needful by approved physicians and surgeons and furnished with the necessary medicines in all diseases except the pox, midwifery, and cutting for stone."

Chamberlain's plan got nowhere, but some 80 years later, in 1769, the British county of Devon instituted its own system of social medical insurance. The effort became an abrupt failure. A report on the experiment concluded: "The gentlemen of the County, finding the financial burden of the poor to increase rapidly, were without any further consideration in a mighty hurry to get the act repealed."

But Britain was changing. By the mid-1800s, 4,000 British doctors were on the government payroll, caring for four million patients. "To those who could perceive it," writes Professor Terence Davies, "socialized medicine had arrived. . . ."

In 1854, Prussia enacted Europe's first large-scale compulsory health insurance law, later expanded into a national program when Bismarck attempted to curb the growing power of German Socialists "by making many features of the Socialist program his own." Part of the Socialist program adopted by Bismarck was a comprehensive national health insurance plan, enacted in 1883.

In 1909, Beatrice Webb, a founder of Britain's Fabian Socialist movement, advocated "a State medical service in which all doctors would be salaried civil servants," a plan similar to the one finally adopted by the British in 1948. The Webb plan was defeated, but in 1911, Lloyd George, who had visited Germany to study the Bismarck plan, pushed through Britain's first program of national health insurance. (Compared to later plans, the first effort was small: approximately one-third of the British workers were covered, and none of their dependents. The plan covered neither hospitalization nor specialist services; but it was a start.)

By the early twentieth century all the countries of continental Europe had adopted social insurance programs, and the idea had spread to America. Federal and state labor bureaus had begun to study the European plans in the 1890s. By 1906, American liberals had banded together in the American Association for Labor Legislation (AALL), organizer of the first major drive for national health insurance in the United States.

The campaign began in earnest immediately after passage of the British program in 1911. That same year, Louis D. Brandeis, later to become a Supreme Court Justice, delivered a ringing speech calling for national health insurance. In 1912, liberal former-President Theodore Roosevelt, running for re-election on the ticket of the new Progressive Party, became the first American presidential candidate to endorse the concept of national health insurance, and saw to it that the plan was written into his party's platform.

Meanwhile, the AALL established a Social-Insurance Committee and summoned the nation's liberals to a "First American Confer-

ence on Social Insurance," held in Chicago, under AALL sponsorship, in 1913. That same year, I. M. Rubinow, a member of the
AALL, published a 500-page book entitled *Social Insurance,* the
textbook for the campaign that was to follow. By 1915, the AALL
had produced a standard health insurance bill and began intensive
lobbying efforts to get government health programs enacted in the
various states.

For two years the campaign flourished. By 1917, the standard bill
had been introduced in 12 state legislatures and eight had appointed study commissions. The nation's most prominent liberals—
Theodore Roosevelt, Governors Samuel McCall of Massachusetts
and Hiram Johnson of California, and Idaho Senator William Borah
—all came out for government health insurance programs.

But the tide turned. As long as the campaign consisted only of
rhetoric, the advocates of government medicine had basked in
success, but when the bills were introduced the voter had a chance
actually to see what it was that was being proposed, and to analyze
the effects of government medicine on medical care and on his
pocketbook.

An aroused public began to clamor against the plan. State legislative study commissions began to return unfavorable reports. When
the voters were given a chance to express themselves, in a California referendum in 1918, government health insurance was overwhelmingly defeated (by a margin of two to one).

In April, 1919, the New York State Assembly decisively defeated an attempt to remove the bill from committee.

The first major effort to adopt government health programs in
the U.S. collapsed in utter failure, rejected by the voters and the
legislatures. Not a single state adopted the proposal. Samuel Gompers, the prestigious president of the American Federation of Labor
and generally considered the founder of the labor movement in the
U.S., resigned from the AALL in protest over its government
health schemes.

The movement for government health insurance in the U.S. was
not revived for nearly a decade. Most of the social activists of the
day turned to other areas in which to work their reforms, but the
1920s were tough years for those who would change the system,
and eventually efforts turned inward—to preparing and waiting.

But if no drastic changes were taking place, the era was what historian Clarke Chambers called "a seedtime of reform." A host of organizations, such as the American Association for Labor Legislation, the American Association of Social Workers, and the National Conference of Social Work, turned their attention to laying the groundwork for new fights in the future. Though today's advocates of national health insurance insist that their desires for change are largely the result of a sudden surge of medical costs, the propaganda campaign against medical costs began nearly half a century ago and has continued since as an essential part of the planners' strategy. Part of the groundwork was laid in 1927, when a handful of the plan's supporters created a political front group, known as the Committee on the Costs of Medical Care.

Ironically, the committee's first effort didn't pan out quite the way its instigators had hoped. When the final report was issued after a five-year study, the committee did *not* recommend national health insurance; to the contrary, a majority of the committee members had decided they preferred *private* insurance. The committee concluded, among other things, "that a private system would be philosophically preferable in a nation that prided itself on freedom and private enterprise."

Then came the depression and Franklin D. Roosevelt.

Just as the hardships of World War II were later to make the British people eager for change, the depression did the same thing to the American people. Roosevelt began to preach an activist role for government and in June, 1934, created a special cabinet "Committee on Economic Security," instructed to explore "all forms of social insurance."

Harry Hopkins, one of Roosevelt's inner circle, pressed the President to give health insurance top priority, as did Rexford Tugwell and Josephine Roche, two members of the special committee, but Frances Perkins, Roosevelt's Labor Secretary, urged that top priority be given to unemployment insurance, instead, and won the support of the American Association for Labor Legislation, which was not eager for a rematch on health insurance.

Roosevelt, concerned that the rest of his program would go down the drain in a fight over health insurance, reluctantly decided to avoid the issue.

Advocates of national health insurance began to press Roosevelt again after the Social Security Act had been safely enacted in August, 1935, but 1936 was an election year and the President was afraid to test the issue in a public vote. He informed Secretary Perkins that he wanted no action in the Congress until the elections were out of the way. (Edwin E. Witte, executive director of the special cabinet Committee on Economic Security, had written a letter in April, 1935, to Edgar Sydenstricker, a committee aide and former member of the Committee on the Costs of Medical Care, in which Witte commented that there did not appear to be "sufficient public interest" to enact a government health insurance program. He had urged an "educational" campaign.)

Roosevelt had not completely shelved the program, though. The day after the Social Security Act was signed, he created an Interdepartmental Committee to Coordinate Health and Welfare Activities, headed by Josephine Roche, one of the strongest advocates of a high-priority health insurance push by the administration. According to the Department of Health, Education and Welfare's 1969 report on "The Evolution of Medicare," the Interdepartmental Committee became the "focal point" of leadership in the drive for national health insurance during the next few years.

Immediately, health insurance became one of the day's major political topics. According to the HEW booklet, "Advocates made numerous public speeches; articles appeared in magazines and journals of every description; and, by 1938, some 15 books had been published on the subject." Support came from a wide spectrum of sources on the political Left, including the Communist Party. William Z. Foster, national chairman of the Communist Party, U.S.A., writing in his book *Toward a Soviet America* (1932), urged a system of social insurance including free medical care.

In 1935 and 1936 the Federal Government directed a National Health Survey that, in its report, claimed among other things that the infant mortality rate in the U.S. exceeded that of any other civilized country. (Today, nearly 40 years later, advocates of national health insurance still use the infant mortality argument to claim that the nation has plunged into a health care "crisis.")

The few faces in the drive for national health insurance began to reappear in overlapping roles. Michael M. Davis, who had been a member of the Committee on the Costs of Medical Care, now established a Committee on Research in Medical Economics to publicize health issues. The American Association for Social

Security, headed by Abraham Epstein, began to lobby for government health insurance. (Epstein drafted a bill which Senator Arthur Capper, of Kansas, introduced in 1935, but the bill received little support.) I.S. Falk, first a member of AALL, then a member of the Committee on the Costs of Medical Care, now showed up as a member of a Technical Committee on Medical Care, set up by Josephine Roche's Interdepartmental Committee.

In the summer of 1937, Miss Roche and Harry Hopkins met privately with half a dozen other advocates of government medicine and decided to formulate a comprehensive national health program. The task of drafting the legislation fell to Falk and the government's Technical Committee on Medical Care.

But one of the major ingredients for success was still missing: the active support of the President.

Roosevelt was urged to raise the issue in the 1938 Congressional elections, but refused. Violent strikes were rocking the New Deal and Roosevelt had suffered a series of major defeats in recent months. The voters had supported anti-New Deal Democrats in the 1938 party primaries, and the economy was in another recession, with nine million people out of work nearly 10 years after the stock market crash. The President was in no mood to take on another hot potato, especially since he secretly intended to seek an unprecedented third term just two years later.

The voters solidly rejected the New Deal in the 1938 general elections. William E. Leuchtenberg, in his book *Franklin D. Roosevelt and the New Deal,* described the election results as "disastrous" for the social planners.

Roosevelt cautiously advised Congress to "study" the national health issue, but in January, 1939, Senator Robert F. Wagner of New York announced that he would introduce his own bill to create a National Health Program. The bill, introduced on February 28 (S. 1620), became the first major piece of legislation aimed at creating national health insurance in the United States. Organized labor took the lead in supporting the Wagner bill, but opposition was intense and the Senate tabled the plan for "further study."

Then came the war. Just as the depression had revived the campaign for national health insurance, the advent of World War II again forestalled it. Roosevelt's attention, and the nation's, turned to the marching armies of Adolf Hitler, Benito Mussolini, and the

Japanese war lords. Domestic legislation took a back seat. The Wagner bill died in committee.

Despite the war, and the public concern with other, more important, matters, the advocates of government medical controls kept working. They knew their chance would come again; during the war years they busied themselves preparing for another round. (Representative Thomas Eliot of Massachusetts introduced a national health insurance proposal in 1942, but it received little attention.)

By 1943, the tide had turned. The Marines and Navy were island-hopping across the Pacific, driving the Japanese back. Allied air power had taken a heavy toll on Nazi war machinery and Hitler had reached a standstill. Gradually, thoughts turned again to domestic schemes.

In his State of the Union message for 1943, President Roosevelt called for a social insurance system that would extend "from the cradle to the grave." In June of that year Senators Wagner and James Murray, of Montana, along with Representative John Dingell, of Michigan, introduced a bill drafted by the Social Security Board that would have added health insurance coverage to the Social Security program.

The Wagner-Murray-Dingell bill signaled the beginning of a major new drive for government medicine. Again the opposition mounted, and again Roosevelt backed off from an all-out endorsement. The bill died in committee; but it would be back.

Finally, Roosevelt decided the time was ripe for an all-out campaign. With the Allied war effort gaining major victories, he enjoyed new popularity. In the election campaign of 1944, which brought him his fourth term as President, Roosevelt called for new health care programs; in his budget message of January, 1945, he called for an extended program of social security, "including medical care"; the Social Security Board drafted a special presidential message on health.

Then, in April, Roosevelt died.

The new President, Harry Truman, jumped immediately into the lists. On November 19, 1945, with the war over, Truman sent a new health message to the Congress, including a revised Wagner-Murray-Dingell bill. For the first time, Congress had before it an official administration proposal for national health insurance.

Truman's open advocacy launched a major new campaign for a national health program. Beginning in 1945, the social planners introduced health insurance proposals into many state legislatures. But the people still wanted no part of the programs; every one of the state proposals was defeated. On Capitol Hill, the bill's backers met a cool response.

Determined to give the public this legislation which it seemed so intent on resisting, the program's backers began a new "education" campaign. Michael Davis, formerly of the Committee on the Costs of Medical Care and the Committee on Research in Medical Economics, now launched a new front to support the Wagner-Murray-Dingell bill—the Committee for the Nation's Health. The American Association for Labor Legislation had folded in 1942, but with Samuel Gompers out of the way the powerful American Federation of Labor now began to push actively for national health programs, working primarily through Davis' committee.

In 1938, the voters had solidly rejected the New Deal programs. In 1946, the first election since 1938 in which domestic issues held the spotlight, the public again rejected the programs. The new Congress wanted no part of President Truman's proposed government takeover of medicine. What's more, the public had become aroused against labor union activities and the powerful labor organizations that had spearheaded the campaign for national health insurance suddenly found themselves fighting against proposed new restrictions on their own "organizing" activities.

In the meantime, the Cold War had begun in earnest: Czechoslovakia fell to the Russians and Red troops blockaded Berlin. Again, as had been the case at the outbreak of World War II, other issues forced national health insurance onto a back burner.

In early 1948, Truman was quoted as saying, reluctantly, that a government health system would probably have to be considered an "ultimate aim" rather than a possibility for the near future. In his State of the Union speech that year Truman markedly omitted any call for national health insurance.

Truman was apparently a man marked for defeat. Even his most enthusiastic supporters conceded there was little chance that Truman would be returned to the White House. With his defeat, the fate of national health insurance would be wrapped in a new question mark, "President" Thomas E. Dewey.

Truman's blistering campaign that year was aimed largely at the
Republican Congress that had opposed his programs. When, surprisingly, he won re-election, advocates of national health insurance immediately declared that the vote had been a mandate for
enactment of the program. (In retrospect, however, most political
historians concluded that the Truman victory was the result of a
vote for the status quo, not a vote for change—and, in large part,
a vote for Truman himself, the spunky small-town Missourian spar-
ring fiercely with the reserved New York lawyer. Health insurance
had not been a key issue.)

When Congress assembled after the 1948 voting, it found that
the resistance to government medicine was even stronger than
before. Labor organizations, pushing at local levels for private
health insurance coverage for their members, had noticeably
cooled in their campaign for government medicine. Within a year,
nearly 2,000 organizations, ranging from the American Bar Association to the General Federation of Women's Clubs, joined in
fighting the program.

By the time the 1950 elections rolled around, liberal incumbents
were visibly shying away from advocacy of national health insurance. Two of the issue's most outspoken advocates, Senators Claude
Pepper, of Florida, and Frank Graham, of North Carolina, were
defeated in party primaries. In the general elections, four more
leading advocates—Senators Elbert Thomas, of Utah, and Glen H.
Taylor, of Idaho, and Representatives Andrew Biemiller, of Wisconsin, and Eugene O'Sullivan, of Nebraska—were defeated.

Temporarily, national health insurance was dead. Truman again
omitted the proposal from his State of the Union speech in 1952.
In the 1952 elections, Adlai Stevenson, the Democratic heir apparent, stayed away from the issue. His Republican opponent, Dwight
D. Eisenhower, came out strongly against the program.

In England, meanwhile, Socialist leaders had enacted a comprehensive new health service, covering every inhabitant of the British
Isles. Doctors had become civil servants on a fixed government
salary. The new law nationalized all the nation's hospitals and permitted the government to confiscate their endowments and transfer
them to a State fund. Doctors who had invested huge sums in their
practices were forbidden, under threat of possible imprisonment,
to buy or sell practices. Advocates of socialized medicine had finally

won a complete victory in England. At about the same time (in 1946) the French government had pushed through a massive cradle-to-grave social security system, partly socializing medical care in that country. In the United States, however, President Eisenhower's election effectively derailed national health insurance for nearly two decades.

It finally became clear to the planners—after more than half a century of frustration and defeat—that the American people were firmly opposed to junking the medical system under which they had fared so well. Yet the advocates of national health insurance remained determined that the people should have such a program, want it or not. Obviously a new approach was called for. If the public would not *knowingly* accept national health insurance, perhaps it could be persuaded to move *unknowingly* toward such a goal.

In 1944, Merrill G. Murray of the Social Security Administration proposed that the advocates of national health insurance consider pushing for a limited program, aimed at the elderly, as "a beginning." After the 1950 elections, when it was clear that the Wagner-Murray-Dingell bill was stalled, the proposed change in tactics won new attention.

I. S. Falk, who had now become the head of the Social Security Administration's Bureau of Research and Statistics, drafted a plan to create a government health insurance program limited to Social Security beneficiaries. Falk's plan became the forerunner of Medicare. According to a 1969 report by Falk's bureau, the planners believed "The proposal would establish the health insurance principle and enable the government to gain experience in this field." And, the report pointed out, focusing such a program on the aged "would enhance the possibilities of enactment."

Robert J. Myers, chief actuary of the Social Security Administration for 23 years, beginning in Truman's first term, described the strategy in a 1969 speech before the American Enterprise Institute:

". . . the ultimate goal of the expansionists is a relatively simple, but comprehensive, one—to provide Medicare benefits for the entire working and retired populations and their dependents . . .

". . . the expansionists would take the gradual approach to their desired social goal. This would be done by first expanding Medicare to some or all of the persons under 65 who are receiving cash benefits. Then, there might be instituted the so-called Kiddicare proposal . . . all financed through Medicare.

". . . This would be another step toward the attainment of the expansionist social goal of nationalizing medical care."

Myers then described how each step would be used to condition the public for the next expansion:

"Certainly the consequence of establishing a Kiddicare program would be to reduce further the potential scope of private insurance. As a result, the relative operating costs of private insurance for the limited benefit area in which it would operate would become high. Private insurance would thus be subject to adverse criticism, and it would be suggested that the governmental plan might as well take over the entire load . . ."

As soon as the decision to switch tactics had been reached, strange coincidences occurred. At the end of February, 1952, Federal Security Administrator Oscar Ewing publicly called for enactment of a national health insurance program limited to Social Security beneficiaries. A little more than a month later, in April, the annual report of the Social Security Administration urged the same program. The same month, Senator Murray and Representative Dingell, joined by two new campaigners, Senator Hubert Humphrey, of Minnesota, and Representative Emanuel Celler, of New York, introduced bills in the Senate and House calling for enactment of the plan into law. In December, President Truman's Commission on the Health Needs of the Nation issued its report—a call for the same program.

As the *New York Times* noted, there was little chance for action in that session of Congress. The liberals who had supported national health programs had suffered heavy losses and Congress was in no mood to tackle the program again. Soon Eisenhower would move into the White House, pledged to oppose the schemes for government medicine. But the "expansionists," as Myers was to call them, had confidence in their new strategy and were content to wait.

In 1956, the planners got some major breaks:

Members of the military service had long been cared for by the government. But in 1956, Congress extended government health services to the dependents of servicemen under the so-called military "Medicare" law. The bill set a precedent that delighted the advocates of Medicare and national health insurance: for the first time, citizens who were neither in the military nor on welfare were to receive medical care through government programs. It was a major breakthrough.

The same Congress played into the hands of the expansionists by authorizing a study of "the problems of the aged." Though the study was not intended to further the campaign for government medicine, the Senate's Special Committee on Aging soon became a forum for the advocates of such programs.

Early the next year, the AFL-CIO Executive Council voted to support the national health insurance campaign with funds drawn from its 14 million members. From that point on, organized labor has dominated the movement to dismantle the private medical system, and national health insurance became labor's top legislative goal. The AFL-CIO persuaded Congressman Aime J. Forand, of Rhode Island, to introduce a Medicare program in the House near the end of the 1957 session. The next year labor conducted an intensive nationwide campaign in behalf of liberal Congressional candidates, delivering a number of new supporters for the Forand bill.

By the time the 1960 Congress opened, the campaign was in full swing. All of the major contenders for the Democratic presidential nomination had come out for a Medicare program, and liberals in the Republican ranks—led by HEW Secretary Arthur Flemming and New York Senator Jacob Javits—pushed for a measure of their own.

In March, 1960, Medicare supporters "won" another defeat: though the House Ways and Means Committee rejected the Forand bill by a two-to-one margin (the actual vote was 17 to 8), the showdown represented the first time the issue had ever reached a formal vote in the committee. The plan's backers seemed to be following the Spanish maxim: "poco a poco, se va lejos"—little by little, one goes a long way.

The bill's supporters continued to mount pressure, using the Senate Subcommittee on Problems of the Aged and Aging as a forum for news coverage; conducting mass public rallies; whipping up "write your Congressman" campaigns. House Speaker Sam Rayburn and Senate Majority Leader Lyndon Johnson came out for Medicare.

Forand forced his bill to another vote in the Ways and Means

Committee. It lost again, by the same count, but Congress, unwilling to accept either Forand's bill or substitutes backed by Flemming, had become willing to accept a compromise—if one could be found. The long campaign had begun to pay off; where Congress had once flatly rejected national health plans, considering each "no" vote a final action, it now considered each "no" vote only a stalemate. It was becoming increasingly certain that half a century of pressure would win for the social planners at least some limited form of national health program, if only to get the advocates off Congressional backs.

Wilbur Mills of Arkansas, chairman of the House Ways and Means Committee, came up with the compromise the Congress could live with: expansion of medical-care payments under state welfare programs to include persons who classified as "medically indigent," but who did not qualify for the various state welfare programs. In the Senate, Oklahoma's Robert S. Kerr put his considerable power behind the Mills plan.

The Kerr-Mills bill was quickly passed by a tired and relieved House. In the Senate, Medicare backers continued to seek "a whole loave," but to no avail. A government health insurance plan, offered as an amendment to Kerr-Mills by Senators John F. Kennedy, of Massachusetts, and Clinton P. Anderson, of New Mexico, was defeated on the Senate floor. Like the House, the Senate passed the Kerr-Mills "compromise" and on September 13, 1960, the President signed the act into law (Public Law 86–778), the first major government medical program.

Kerr-Mills (later to become Medicaid) did not end the fight, however. Although the plan's backers hoped the advocates of national health insurance would be satisfied with the major victory they had achieved, such was not the case. Even Medicare itself, whenever it was accomplished, was only to be "a beginning." As Robert Myers had said: "This would be *another step* toward the attainment of the expansionist social goal of nationalizing medical care."

The same year that the Kerr-Mills bill was enacted, John F. Kennedy campaigned for president on a platform that included Medicare. When he was elected, the backers of a government health insurance program suddenly could count on White House backing again, for the first time in nearly a decade.

The campaign began in earnest once more. President-elect Kennedy appointed a Special Task Force on Health and Social Security for the American People, headed by Medicare advocate Wilbur J. Cohen, later to become Lyndon Johnson's Secretary of Health, Education and Welfare. (Not surprisingly, the committee recommended hospital insurance under Social Security.) Kennedy then appointed Cohen to serve as Assistant Secretary for Legislation at HEW, in charge of the administration's campaign for the adoption of Medicare.

Soon after he took office, Kennedy sent his health insurance bill to Congress, authored by Senator Anderson and Representative Cecil King, of California. But government health insurance, now closer than ever before, was, it seemed, as far away as ever. Kennedy's victory margin had been the smallest in recent history. Not only did he not have a "mandate," his party had lost 20 seats in the House and picked up only two in the Senate. Even with White House support, there were simply not enough votes in Congress for the King-Anderson bill. Stopped again, after 50 years of campaigning, the planners waited for the 1962 elections when, they hoped, Kennedy would win the backing he—and they—needed.

In the meantime, as the bill's opponents fought desperately to prevent government medicine, the AFL-CIO mobilized local pressure groups in the home districts of the Congressmen sitting on the House Ways and Means Committee.

Although the Social Security Administration has reported that a vast majority of the nation's physicians opposed government health programs, arguing that such plans had decreased the quality of medical care and increased health costs in other countries, a small group of doctors, including Benjamin Spock, organized as a "Physician's Committee for Health Care Through Social Security."

Retired Congressman Forand, author of a Medicare bill of his own a few years before, now turned a Kennedy campaign organization (Senior Citizens for Kennedy) into a new front group, The National Council of Senior Citizens for Health Care Through Social Security, with a membership nucleus drawn from organizations of retired union members, including groups set up by the United Auto Workers, United Steel Workers, and International Ladies' Garment Workers.

As the 1962 Congressional elections drew nearer, HEW Secretary Abraham Ribicoff pledged "a great fight across the land" for Medicare. The White House set up 14 regional conferences that stressed the campaign for Medicare. On May 20, 1962, President Kennedy delivered a national television speech calling for the passage of Medicare, while other spokesmen delivered similar speeches in 45 cities across the country. A spokesman for the American Medical Association complained that the administration was conducting a "propaganda blitz" to pressure Congressmen. The Treasury, he said, was being "looted" to finance a massive lobbying campaign.

There was still not enough support to bring the bill to a vote in the House, but an agreement between Anderson and Javits on a Medicare compromise encouraged the bill's supporters to seek a vote in the Senate. A vote on the Anderson-Javits amendment failed, 52–48.

Several factors contributed to the fact that the amendment was defeated despite the major nationwide campaign by the administration. For one thing, a televised rebuttal to Kennedy's speech by Dr. Edward Annis of the American Medical Association brought a flood of mail into Congress, bitterly opposing the government health scheme. Polls showed the President's popularity sagging. Congress had dealt Kennedy a string of defeats. Former President Eisenhower said the whole Kennedy administration was "floundering." Syndicated columnist Walter Lippmann wrote that there was just not any great compulsion for the proposals Kennedy was advocating.

The 1962 elections arrived with Medicare still a question mark. However, Kennedy's handling of the Cuban missile crisis won general public support just before the election and brought four new administration supporters to the Senate (which, coupled with the death of Kerr, almost assured Senate passage of Medicare).

Then, in November, 1963, as the Kennedy administration turned to the Medicare issue again, the President was murdered. "One of the many consequences of that tragedy," reported the Social Security Administration, "was a surge of public support for the martyred President's legislative program. The new President moved quickly to act upon these sentiments. Mr. Johnson began exhorting Congress to act on all manner of issues, including Medicare."

Although there was still not enough support to pass a Medicare bill in the House (Kennedy had actually lost strength there in the 1962 elections), supporters of government health insurance won a major victory when the Senate finally voted 49–44 to pass King-Anderson as an amendment to a bill increasing Social Security benefits. The bill died in a deadlocked House-Senate conference committee, but the plan's backers had again moved one step closer.

The big break came in 1964 when President Johnson won a landslide presidential victory over Republican Senator Barry Goldwater. Johnson resumed his office in January, 1965, with comfortable majorities in both houses of Congress. The King-Anderson bill was quickly reintroduced in both houses. On March 23, 1965, the House Ways and Means Committee substituted a revised bill, drafted by Chairman Wilbur Mills, and on April 8, after a single day of debate, the bill was passed. On July 9, the bill was passed by the Senate. A conference committee report was approved by both houses before the end of the month.

When Lyndon Johnson signed the Medicare bill into law, the backers of national health insurance had at last accomplished the first step toward their goal.

And Medicare was to be just that: a first step.

Immediately after the plan was adopted, a new campaign began —this time for a total national health program.

Appendix II.
The Planners' Plans

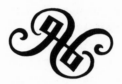

If the United States adopts an expanded government health care system, it will probably come in the form of one of these plans (or some revised version of them):

HEALTH SECURITY ACT (S. 3, H.R. 22)—The Kennedy-Reuther bill.

Sponsor: Introduced by Senator Edward M. Kennedy and Representative Martha Griffiths. Drafted by the Committee for National Health Insurance, headed by the late Walter Reuther and now by his successor as UAW president, Leonard Woodcock. Committee members include Senators Kennedy and John Sherman Cooper; former Senators Paul Douglas and Ralph Yarborough; Reverend Ralph Abernathy of the Southern Christian Leadership Conference and Mrs. Martin Luther King, the widow of his predecessor; Arthur Goldberg; John Kenneth Galbraith; General James M. Gavin; former University of California Chancellor Clark Kerr; former Cleveland Mayor Carl Stokes. Senator Edmund Muskie is a co-sponsor of the bill. The bill combines the original Kennedy bill with features of a bill introduced in 1970 by Representative Griffiths, with the backing of the AFL-CIO.

Provisions: The program would be compulsory for all Americans and would provide comprehensive health benefits (except dental care for adults, which would be added later). It would provide unlimited coverage for physician visits and care (including surgery) and for hospital care; hospital psychiatric care (with a 45-day limit); skilled nursing-home care (120-day limit per spell of illness); up to 20 visits (per spell of illness) to a fee-for-service physician for psychiatric care. The program would pay most of the cost, but not all, for eye glasses, appliances (braces, artificial limbs, etc.), laboratory services, podiatry, optometry, ambulance services, physiotherapy and home health services.

The bill would eliminate private insurance plans (which now cover some 170 million persons, or 85 percent of the population).

The Kennedy-Griffiths bill, as originally introduced, would allocate two to five percent of the funds available under the program for development of group pre-payment plans. Fee-for-service practice would be allowed under the law, but payment schedules are strongly weighted to discourage such a manner of practice. For example, all prescribed drugs would be covered in full by the plan's benefits if prescribed by a doctor in a group pre-payment plan, but only maintenance drugs would be covered if prescribed by a private physician practicing by the traditional fee-for-service method.

The group-plan concept is further promoted by the payment provisions of the law: Benefits will be paid first to institutional providers of care (including hospitals and clinics), and then to pre-payment group practices and fee-for-service practitioners. (Fee-for-service merely means that a patient pays a doctor for each treatment, when rendered, rather than in a pre-arranged annual sum.) Pre-payment group physicians and fee-for-service physicians would be paid a proportionate share of their fees, based on comprehensiveness of service. Thus a large group would receive a larger payment for each patient than would an individual physician.

The Department of Health, Education and Welfare estimates the first year costs of the Kennedy program at $77 billion. Robert J. Myers, chief actuary of HEW's Social Security Administration for 23 years, has computed that income for that first year (1974) will total approximately $57 billion—or $20 billion less than expenses. According to the payment provisions, then, institutions would be paid for their services to patients; bills submitted by fee-for-service practitioners for their services would likely remain unpaid or be paid only in small part, since private practitioners are to receive only what is left after the institutions have been paid. (Obviously such a program will effectively force most physicians into large group plans or out of practice entirely. The provision is based on a belief that group pre-payment plans will increase efficiency by concentrating many physician and clinical services under a single roof. But the plan has several serious drawbacks, discussed in Chapter 7.)

According to the proposal, advance budgets would be drawn up for each of the nation's health care "regions," and spending within each region would be limited in accordance with the budget. Thus, hospitals, clinics, physicians, dentists, pharmacists and suppliers of medical devices (eyeglasses, dental braces, etc.) would be paid only to the extent to which previously budgeted funds were available. (If administering bureaucrats were to misgauge public demand for a service, or if they found it advantageous to report "reduced health care costs" in their regions—possibly to obtain favorable notice at headquarters—physicians might find themselves working for free, or for a small percentage of their earned fees.)

In his introduction to Daniel Schorr's book *Don't Get Sick In America,* Senator Kennedy called repeatedly for a "revolution" that would result in a new system of providing medical care. This bill would move in that direction by creating a Resources Development Fund to initiate studies and projects aimed at complete reorganization of the present care system. So-called "consumer" groups— primarily liberal "front" organizations, consisting almost exclusively of non-physicians—would be given a major role in establishing health care programs.

The bill would create a separate bureaucracy, consisting of a National Health Security Board, with regional and local overseers.

Costs: Approximately 36 percent of the estimated income would come from payroll taxes, paid by employers on their total payrolls, with no maximum taxable-earnings base; 12 percent would come from direct individual payroll taxes; two percent would come from taxes on the self-employed; 50 percent would come from general tax revenues. The employer payroll tax would be at a rate of 3.5 percent, the self-employed tax at a rate of 2.5 percent, the individual tax at a rate of 1.0 percent on income up to $15,000.

According to the bill's supporters, the maximum direct individual payroll tax under the original bill would have been $315 a year, for top income brackets. That, however, is only a small part of the story.

The individual wage earner must also pay the increased taxes to provide the 50 percent that is to come from general revenues. What is more, the employee pays indirectly, in reduced salary, for the amount paid by his employer. Myers' actuarial studies for the Social Security Administration indicated an actual annual average cost of $660 a year from each worker (not $315). What is more, if income is increased (as it was with Medicare) to meet the costs estimated by HEW, each worker will contribute about one-third more—or nearly $1,000 a year.

The remainder of the bills introduced so far are wholly or partially voluntary. They include:

NATIONAL HEALTH INSURANCE PARTNERSHIP, FAMILY HEALTH INSURANCE PLAN and other proposals—The Nixon Plan.

Sponsor: The official program of the Nixon Administration, outlined in a Presidential message to the Congress on February 18, 1971.

Provisions: The first section of the program would create a "National Health Insurance Partnership" plan (NHIP) under which employers would be required to provide comprehensive health insurance for their employees. Minimum benefits would include hospital and physician care, full maternity care, well-baby care, laboratory services, and a minimum of $50,000 in "catastrophic illness" coverage for physician fees and hospital charges. Employers would buy the insurance from private companies and would be required to pay at least 65 percent of the cost for the first 30 months and 75 percent thereafter, with the employee paying the remaining portion.

Employees may choose to enroll in a Health Maintenance Organization (pre-paid group practice) rather than receive private insurance coverage.

Employers would be compelled to offer the health insurance coverage but employee acceptance of the offer (including the employee's commitment to pay the remaining 25–35 percent of the premium cost) would be voluntary.

The program would go into effect on July 1, 1973.

The second portion of the Nixon health program provides a

Family Health Insurance Plan (FHIP) under which taxpayers would buy basic medical coverage for the medically indigent (income of $5,000 or less for a family of four). Families with an income of $3,000 or less would receive all medical and health care free; families with incomes between $3,000 and $5,000 would pay part of the costs through a graduated schedule of premiums, deductibles and coinsurance.

The plan would be completely administered and financed by the Federal Government. It would replace Title 19 of the Social Security Act (Medicaid) that is administered by state governments and financed by the state and Federal governments.

The third portion of the program would use loans and grants to encourage the formation of Health Maintenance Organizations (large pre-payment groups). The administration has announced a goal of having 90 percent of the population treated in such groups by 1980.

The final portion of the program deals with Federal grants and loans to encourage medical personnel to move into rural areas or run-down sections of large cities. It would also provide grants to medical schools based on the number of doctors graduated each year.

Costs: Estimated at $12.4 billion.

THE MINIMUM HEALTH BENEFITS AND SERVICES DISTRIBUTION AND EDUCATION ACT (S. 703).

Sponsor: Introduced by Senator Claiborne Pell (D-Rhode Island).

Provisions: Like the Nixon plan, Senator Pell's program would require employers to provide a minimum level of health benefits to their employees. The bill specifies these annual benefits: One complete diagnostic examination; visits to physician, out-patient clinic or other ambulatory health care facility which are necessary for the treatment of illness or injury, or to prevent illness or injury; up to 12 days of hospital care (after two days paid by the insured); up to 10 days of care in an extended-care unit for recovery from serious illness, accident or surgery; emergency room service; maternity benefits, including pre-natal care; preventive care by physicians; care of optometrists, podiatrists and chiropractors; therapeutic devices (for example, eyeglasses, hearing aids, etc.) if important to maintain employability; prescription drugs; catastrophic-illness coverage.

The plan also would authorize community health corporations to provide comprehensive health service. (Most states now have laws that prohibit non-physicians from dispensing medical care).

Costs: No cost estimates have been made available.

THE NATIONAL HEALTH INSURANCE AND HEALTH SERVICES IMPROVEMENT ACT (S. 836)—The Javits Bill.

Sponsor: Introduced by Senator Jacob Javits (R-New York). The bill was at least partially drafted for Javits by former HEW Secretary Wilbur Cohen.

Provisions: The Javits bill would in effect extend Medicare to cover all the nation's citizens (it now covers only the elderly). It would first extend coverage to the disabled, unemployed and poor, and would reach full coverage by July 1, 1974. The bill would also add coverage of maintenance drugs, with a $1 fee paid by the patient; physical examinations for all; and dental care for children under eight years of age.

An employee could refuse to participate in the plan if (a) he was covered under an approved alternative plan offered by his employer, provided the employer paid at least 75 percent of the cost, or (b) he was covered under an approved private insurance program.

Costs: Payroll taxes on both employers and employees at a rate of 0.7 percent in 1972, increasing to 3.3 percent by 1976. The Federal Government would contribute an amount equal to one-half of the amount contributed by the employers and employees.

The Social Security Administration has estimated that the program would cost $66.4 billion in 1975 when fully implemented.

THE HEALTH CARE INSURANCE ASSISTANCE ACT (S. 987, H.R. 4960)—"Medicredit."

Sponsors: The bill was introduced in the House by Representatives Richard Fulton (D-Tennessee) and Joel Broyhill (R-Virginia). It is patterned after a "Medicredit Tax Incentive Plan" devised by the American Medical Association and has been endorsed by the AMA.

Provisions: The program would be offered on a voluntary basis to all citizens under 65. Minimum benefits would include physician services, and hospitalization up to 60 days; subject to cost sharing (20 percent coinsurance on the first $500 of medical expense and on the first $500 of emergency or outpatient expense) and deductibles ($50 per hospital stay). Coinsurance and deductibles would be waived for the poor. The program would also provide catastrophic-illness coverage (major medical) after a beneficiary had expended a certain amount above the basic coverage, based on taxable income (10 percent on the first $4,000, 15 percent on the next $3,000, and 20 percent thereafter).

A Federal advisory board would establish standards to be followed by state insurance departments in approving private health insurance plans.

Under the bill, the Federal Government would pay 100 percent of the premium for low-income beneficiaries (an individual and his dependents whose combined annual income would not give rise to any income tax liability). For others the government would provide scaled participation ranging between 10 percent and 99 percent in the payment of premiums for basic coverage, and would pay in full the premiums for catastrophic coverage. The extent of Federal subsidization for each individual would be based on that individual's income tax liability. Persons with higher incomes (thus, higher tax liabilities) would receive less Federal money for health insurance purchases. (In other words, the person who contributes the least to the Federal Government gets the most from it; the person who contributes the most gets the least.)

Costs: The AMA estimates total cost of the program at $12.1 billion in new money; HEW says it would cost $15 billion.

Some medical observers believe the Javits bill stands the best chance of adoption, being most nearly a compromise between Medicredit and the Kennedy-Griffiths plan. Javits may also gain support from the fact that his plan is merely an extension of a familiar and existing program. On the other hand, Medicare has now been so universally recognized as a failure that legislators may not want to follow the same path again.

In addition, there are several other bills in the hopper, each of which may stand a fair chance of adoption when the final Congressional maneuvering begins. Among them:

THE NATIONAL HEALTH CARE ACT (H.R. 4349)—the program of the Health Insurance Association of America, introduced by Representative Omar Burleson (D-Texas), a member of the House Ways and Means Committee.

This bill would make comprehensive private health insurance

policies available to all through a system of Federal income tax credits. Persons unable to purchase or obtain health insurance would be insured through state pools of private health insurers, supported by Federal and state funds through taxes scaled according to income levels.

The bill would establish a minimum standard of health care benefits to be included in all qualified health insurance policies.

Different levels of minimum benefits would be required for (a) private group and individual plans, and (b) the poor and uninsurable. A broader range of benefits would be included in state-paid plans for the poor.

Private group and individual plans would initially cover 30 days of hospital care, 60 days of skilled nursing-home care, 90 days of home health care, X-ray and laboratory services, three visits a year (per family member) to a physician, and well-baby care. *For the poor,* the insurance would cover six visits per year (per family member) to a physician; increased well-baby care, 120 days of hospitalization, 120 days of skilled nursing-home care, and 180 days of home health care, as well as dental care for children under 19, prescription drugs, rehabilitation services and family planning services.

Minimum benefits would be expanded to full coverage by 1979. An employer would be prohibited from showing income tax deductions for employee health care unless he was providing a health care policy meeting the bill's standards. Individuals would be permitted unlimited tax deductions for all the costs of purchasing qualified individual health care policies.

A family of three or four would qualify for the state-paid benefits if the family income did not exceed $6,000 per year. Individuals would qualify if income was less than $3,000 a year.

Representative Burleson has estimated the cost of the program at about $4 billion.

AMERIPLAN—The bill of the American Hospital Association. The plan was drafted by an AHA committee headed by Philadelphia businessman Earl Perloff.

All health resources in an area—physicians, dentists, pharmacists, hospitals, nurses, medical schools, etc.—would be gathered into a single organization to provide comprehensive care to all residents of the area. The organizations—health corporations—would be regulated by new state health commissions and would be financed by government and private funds, with citizens paying according to ability, either directly into the health corporations, through prepaid medical programs, or through private health insurance programs.

Patients would join voluntarily. Physicians and hospitals would be permitted to remain out of the plans, but would be pressured to join by payment methods.

Corporations would provide a standard benefits package, paid in whole for the poor and in part for the near-poor, from general Federal revenues. Services for the aged would be paid from Social Security taxes. Catastrophic-illness coverage would be paid in whole for the poor and in part for the near-poor from general Federal revenues, and for everyone else from Social Security revenues.

ELDERCARE—Proposed by Representative Durward Hall (R-Missouri), a physician. "Eldercare" would provide state-purchased hospitalization policies for the "poor" with the Federal Government reimbursing the states for 85 percent of the premium costs. The policies would be purchased from private companies, including Blue Cross and Blue Shield. States would also provide catastrophic-illness coverage for the poor, with no Federal reimbursement.

The non-poor would pay into a special Social Security fund through increased salary deductions. Persons who do not contribute to Social Security would pay into the fund when they make out income tax returns. The funds in the Social Security pool would provide catastrophic coverage.

Representative Hall has estimated the cost of Part A (the policy for the poor) at $3.7 billion a year in Federal money and $600 million a year in state money. There is no cost estimate available for the provisions for catastrophic coverage for the non-poor.

NATIONAL CATASTROPHIC ILLNESS PROTECTION ACT (H.R. 817)—introduced by Representative Lawrence Hogan, of Massachusetts. This plan would provide for a national program of catastrophic-illness insurance, administered by the states. The Federal Government would provide the program in states that failed to comply.

Risks would be allocated among various insuring companies, and premium rates would be established by the Federal Government.

Premium rates would be lower than customary to encourage purchase of extended health insurance, and the Federal Government (meaning the taxpayers) would compensate insurance companies for losses incurred by them as a result of the lowered premiums.

There are no cost estimates available.

Index